Management of
Esophageal Disasters

Editors

STEPHANIE G. WORRELL
OLUGBENGA T. OKUSANYA

THORACIC
SURGERY CLINICS

www.thoracic.theclinics.com

Consulting Editor
VIRGINIA R. LITLE

November 2024 • Volume 34 • Number 4

ELSEVIER

1600 John F. Kennedy Boulevard • Suite 1800 • Philadelphia, Pennsylvania, 19103-2899

http://www.thoracic.theclinics.com

THORACIC SURGERY CLINICS Volume 34, Number 4
November 2024 ISSN 1547-4127, ISBN-13: 978-0-443-29346-7

Editor: John Vassallo (j.vassallo@elsevier.com)
Developmental Editor: Anita Chamoli

Thoracic Surgery Clinics (ISSN 1547-4127) is published quarterly by Elsevier Inc., 360 Park Avenue South, New York, NY 10010-1710. Months of publication are February, May, August, and November. Business and editorial offices: 1600 John F. Kennedy Boulevard, Suite 1800, Philadelphia, PA 19103-2899. Periodicals postage paid at New York, NY, and additional mailing offices. Subscription prices are $434.00 per year (US individuals), $100.00 per year (US students), $487.00 per year (Canadian individuals), $100.00 per year (Canadian students), $225.00 per year (international students), $524.00 per year (international individuals). For institutional access pricing please contact Customer Service via the contact information below Foreign air speed delivery is included in all Clinics' subscription prices. All prices are subject to change without notice. Orders, claims, and journal inquiries: Please visit our Support Hub page https://service.elsevier.com for assistance.

Reprints. For copies of 100 or more, of articles in this publication, please contact Commercial Rights Department, Elsevier Inc., 360 Park Avenue South, New York, NY 10010-1710. Tel: 212-633-3874; Fax: 212-633-3820; E-mail: reprints@elsevier.com.

Thoracic Surgery Clinics is covered in *MEDLINE/PubMed (Index Medicus), EMBASE/Excerpta Medica, Science Citation Index Expanded (SciSearch®), Journal Citation Reports/Science Edition,* and *Current Contents®/Clinical Medicine.*

Contributors

CONSULTING EDITOR

VIRGINIA R. LITLE, MD
Chief of Thoracic Surgery, Steward Medical
Group Thoracic Surgery, Brighton,
Massachusetts, USA

EDITORS

STEPHANIE G. WORRELL, MD
Section Chief of Thoracic Surgery, Associate
Professor, Department of Surgery, University
of Arizona, Tucson, Arizona

OLUGBENGA T. OKUSANYA, MD
Associate Professor of Surgery, Division of
Thoracic and Esophageal Surgery, Thomas
Jefferson University, Philadelphia,
Pennsylvania

AUTHORS

EVAN T. ALICUBEN, MD
Assistant Professor, Division of Thoracic
Surgery, Department of Cardiothoracic
Surgery, University of Pittsburgh Medical
Center, Pittsburgh, Pennsylvania

SHAHIN AYAZI, MD
Staff Surgeon, Director of Clinical Research,
Foregut Division, Surgical Institute, Allegheny
Health Network Chevalier Jackson Research
Foundation, Director of Clinical Research
Esophageal Institute, Western Pennsylvania
Hospital, Pittsburgh, Pennsylvania;
Department of Surgery, Drexel University,
Philadelphia, Pennsylvania

NICHOLAS BAKER, MD
Assistant Professor, Department of
Cardiothoracic Surgery, University of
Pittsburgh Medical Center, Pittsburgh,
Pennsylvania

SARAH CLIFFORD, BS
MD Candidate, Division of Thoracic Surgery,
Department of Cardiothoracic Surgery,
University of Pittsburgh Medical Center,
Pittsburgh, Pennsylvania

HOPE CONRAD, MD
General Surgery Resident, Thoracic Surgery
Research Fellow, Division of Thoracic Surgery,
Department of Surgery, University of Arizona,
Tucson, Arizona

JULIE M. CORBETT, MD
Esophageal Surgery Fellow, Foregut Division,
Surgical Institute, Allegheny Health Network;
Pittsburgh, Pennsylvania

ANDREW P. DHANASOPON, MD
Assistant Professor, Division of Thoracic
Surgery, Yale School of Medicine, New Haven,
Connecticut

SVEN E. ERIKSSON, MD
Postdoctoral candidate, Foregut Division,
Surgical Institute, Allegheny Health Network;
Chevalier Jackson Research Foundation,
Esophageal Institute, Western Pennsylvania
Hospital, Pittsburgh, Pennsylvania

ERIN ALEXIS GILLASPIE, MD, MPH, FACS
Chief of Thoracic Surgery, Associate Professor
with Tenure, Creighton University Medical
Center, CHI Health, Omaha, Nebraska

JORDAN GREWAL, MD
General Surgery Resident, Vanderbilt University Medical Center, Nashville, Tennessee

SHAWN S. GROTH, MD, MS, FACS
Associate Professor and Chief, Division of Thoracic Surgery, Michael E. DeBakey Department of Surgery, Baylor College of Medicine, Houston, Texas

BLAIR A. JOBE, MD
Director, Foregut Division, Surgical Institute, Allegheny Health Network; Chevalier Jackson Research Foundation, Esophageal Institute, Western Pennsylvania Hospital, Pittsburgh, Pennsylvania; Department of Surgery, Drexel University, Philadelphia, Pennsylvania

COREY KELSOM, PharmD, MS
Scientific Editor, Division of Thoracic Surgery, Department of Cardiothoracic Surgery, University of Pittsburgh Medical Center, Pittsburgh, Pennsylvania

FRANCOIS KHAZOOM, MD, MSc
Fellow, Division of Thoracic Surgery, Swedish Cancer and Digestive Health Institutes at Swedish Medical Center, Seattle, Washington

KELSEY E. KOCH, MD
Fellow, Division of Thoracic Surgery, Yale School of Medicine, New Haven, Connecticut

JOHN C. KUCHARCZUK, MD
Professor of Thoracic Surgery, Department of Surgery, Hospital of the University of Pennsylvania, Philadelphia, Pennsylvania

ADAM H. LACKEY, MD
Thoracic Surgeon, Department of Surgery, Robert Wood Johnson Barnabas Health; Cooperman Barnabas Medical Center, Livingston, New Jersey, USA

KIRAN LAGISETTY, MD
Assistant Professor, Department of Surgery, University of Michigan, Ann Arbor, Michigan

BRIAN E. LOUIE, MD, MPH, MHA, FRCSC, FACS
Executive Medical Director, Division of Thoracic Surgery; Chair, Digestive Health Institute, Swedish Cancer and Digestive Health Institutes at Swedish Medical Center, Seattle, Washington

INANC SAMIL SARICI, MD
Research Fellow, Foregut Division, Surgical Institute, Allegheny Health Network; Chevalier Jackson Research Foundation, Esophageal Institute, Western Pennsylvania Hospital, Pittsburgh, Pennsylvania

LEAH J. SCHOEL, MD
Resident Surgeon, Department of Surgery, University of Michigan, Ann Arbor, Michigan

JOANNA SESTI, MD
Chief, Department of Thoracic Surgery, Northern Region Robert Wood Johnson Barnabas Health, Section Chief, Department of Thoracic Surgery, Cooperman Barnabas Medical Center, Livingston, New Jersey

JACQUELINE M. SOEGAARD BALLESTER, MD, MBMI
General Surgery Resident, Department of Surgery, Hospital of the University of Pennsylvania, Philadelphia, Pennsylvania

PRAVEEN SRIDHAR, MD
Assistant Professor, Division of Thoracic Surgery, Department of Surgery, University of Arizona, Tucson, Arizona

CHRISTOPHER STRADER, MD
Cardiothoracic Surgery Fellow, Division of Thoracic Surgery, Michael E. DeBakey Department of Surgery, Baylor College of Medicine, Houston, Texas

MEGAN TURNER, MD
Resident Physician, Department of Cardiothoracic Surgery, University of Pittsburgh Medical Center, Pittsburgh, Pennsylvania

GAVITT A. WOODARD, MD
Assistant Professor, Division of Thoracic Surgery, Yale School of Medicine, New Haven, Connecticut

Contents

Fistulae between the esophagus and the pericardium or the left atrium are rare but feared complications of transcatheter ablations and esophageal procedures and pathologies. Patients may present variably with cardiopulmonary, gastrointestinal, infectious, and/or neurologic symptoms; a high index of suspicion is paramount. The presence of atrial involvement will dictate the approach and extent of the necessary intervention. While mortality is high overall, surgical repair confers the highest likelihood of survival.

Acquired tracheoesophageal fistulas (TEFs) are rare pathologic connections between the trachea and esophagus. Esophageal and tracheal stenting have been increasingly and safely utilized in management of TEFs, but surgical repair remains the most definitive treatment. Surgical approach to treating TEFs depends on its location, but principles include division and closure of the fistula tracts and insertion of a muscle flap in between the repairs to buttress and prevent recurrence. Advances in diagnostic tools, endoscopic and surgical methods, and intensive care have led to significantly improved outcomes in the management of acquired TEFs.

This article outlines the anatomic and physiologic basis for gastric conduit ischemia and the range of its possible manifestations, from superficial mucosal ischemia to gross conduit necrosis. Methods by which these complications are suspected and ultimately diagnosed are discussed, focusing on clinical and laboratory signs as the harbingers and the use of imaging and endoscopy for confirmation. From there, management options are detailed based on the Esophagectomy Complications Consensus Group classification of esophageal leak and gastric necrosis. Finally, the short- and long-term implications of these complications are reviewed.

THORACIC SURGERY CLINICS

SERIES OF RELATED INTEREST

Advances in Surgery
http://www.advancessurgery.com/

Surgical Clinics
http://www.surgical.theclinics.com/

Surgical Oncology Clinics
https://www.surgonc.theclinics.com/

THE CLINICS ARE AVAILABLE ONLINE!
Access your subscription at:
www.theclinics.com

Foreword
Esophageal Disasters: A Redundant Term?

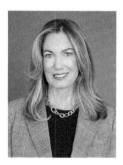

Virginia R. Litle, MD
Consulting Editor

As general thoracic surgeons, we carry out high-risk procedures during which intraoperative deaths are possible—and emotionally painful if they occur. For those of us with busy esophageal practices, disasters can occur preoperatively necessitating urgent and thoughtful use of our skill set. Less often, major problems occur intraoperatively, and more often, they happen postoperatively, where the concern of a bad outcome can linger until the patient is truly on the mend. Guest Editors and Esophagologists Drs Stephanie Worrell and Olugbenga Okusanya produced a list of complicated esophageal scenarios and then potential postoperative problems to lose sleep over. Drs Worrell and Okusanya then invited experts to address these issues from airway esophageal fistulas to iatrogenic perforations to the horrendous esophageal-pericardial, esophageal atrial (EAF), and aorto-esophageal fistulas (AEF). This issue is an excellent summary of caring for a diversity of multiple problems, and we

can take home some management pearls. We learn about fun facts and ideas: ones we know, ones that are unique, and ones that should be investigated.

Starting with five facts we likely know: (1) Endoscopic clipping of perforations can be done for holes less than 1 cm; (2) 30-day mortality from an esophagectomy for a perforated esophageal cancer can reach as high as 63%; (3) Thoracic endovascular aortic repair (TEVAR) alone for an AEF is not definitive therapy (and TEVAR can incite an AEF anyway); (4) The risk of EAF is ∼0.025%, and cryoballoon ablation has a lower fistula rate than radiofrequency ablation per an international study; (5) Asymptomatic reherniation after repair of a paraesophageal hernia on surveillance esophagram is not an instant indication for a reoperation.

Continuing with four unique thoughts: (1) Endoscopic reduction of a paraesophageal hernia and then placing a second scope concurrently for the

Thorac Surg Clin 34 (2024) ix–x
https://doi.org/10.1016/j.thorsurg.2024.07.008
1547-4127/24/© 2024 Published by Elsevier Inc.

percutaneous gastrostomy tube; (2) Tuberculosis can cause an AEF; (3) Median time from atrial ablation to symptoms of fever, chest pain, or neurologic signs from an EAF is 18 days; (4) Patients with spinal deformities (kyphosis, scoliosis) have a higher risk of reherniation after repair.

Several ideas which should be addressed further: (1) Emulsified adipose tissue stromal vascular fracture injection (also known as "cellular therapies") for perforations; (2) When should upper endoscopy be used to evaluate a patient with possible AEF?; (3) Should there be routine endoscopic surveillance after ablation procedures for arrhythmias for early identification of an ulcer? Reading this issue will likely provide more investigative inspiration.

Thank you to Drs Worrell and Okusanya and to *all* the contributors to this Esophageal Disasters issue of *Thoracic Surgery Clinics*, a handbook on the clinical standard of care for identifying and managing challenging foregut issues. These problems keep us on our toes but remain fodder for appreciating how we can benefit our patients. Keep calm and swallow on.

Virginia R. Litle, MD
St. Elizabeth's Medical Center
11 Nevins Street, Suite 201
Brighton, MA 02135, USA

E-mail address:
Vlitle@gmail.com

Twitter: @vlitlemd (V.R. Litle)

Preface

Managing Esophageal Disasters: What to Expect and What to Do

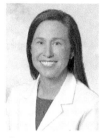 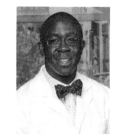

Stephanie G. Worrell, MD   Olugbenga T. Okusanya, MD

Editors

The esophagus has always been a complex organ to manage. Much of the complexity belongs to the location of the esophagus within the posterior mediastinum and the lack of a serosal layer. These two issues make it prone to injury from nearby procedures and challenging to heal when injured or devascularized.

This issue is dedicated to the myriad esophageal disasters many thoracic surgeons encounter. Often, these are only encountered a handful of times in one's career, making consistent and effective treatment algorithms difficult to hone. These articles aim to provide valuable tips on diagnosing, managing, and treating these rare complications.

As our population continues to age, esophageal cancer prevalence continues to rise, and as more patients become long-term survivors of esophageal cancer, it is likely that more complex and challenging scenarios will unfold for those who treat esophageal disease. The wide range of possibilities of esophageal disease that thoracic surgeons must be prepared for will continue to broaden.

The key takeaway messages are consistent throughout each topic. Operation on the esophagus, whether it be a benign paraesophageal hernia or a malignant esophageal cancer, remains a technically complex operation in a challenging patient population. Injuries that occur either during an operation or spontaneously are best managed expeditiously to decrease the morbidity and mortality associated with these devastating problems. Endoscopy continues to play an essential and more prominent role in the treatment of complications for a variety of esophageal operations and issues, including paraesophageal hernia repair, per-oral endoscopic myotomy, trachea-esophageal fistula, and iatrogenic perforations. With continued endoscopic advances, our therapeutic operations for esophageal disasters will likely continue to evolve. These newer approaches will hopefully minimize the morbidity and mortality associated with esophageal disasters.

Esophageal disasters, although rare, are increasing in incidence. As thoracic surgeons, we must be aware of these possible scenarios and have a well-thought-out treatment plan for these complex patients. This issue aims to aid in that effort.

Thorac Surg Clin 34 (2024) xi–xii
https://doi.org/10.1016/j.thorsurg.2024.07.003
1547-4127/24/© 2024 Published by Elsevier Inc.

DISCLOSURES

S.G. Worrell: Speaker for Intuitive; O.T. Okusanya: Speaker for Intuitive and Johnson & Johnson.

FUNDING

No funding.

Stephanie G. Worrell, MD
Department of Surgery
University of Arizona
1501 North Campbell Avenue
Tucson, AZ 85724, USA

Olugbenga T. Okusanya, MD
Division of Thoracic and Esophageal Surgery
Thomas Jefferson University
Philadelphia, PA, USA

E-mail addresses:
sworrell@arizona.edu (S.G. Worrell)
olugbenga.okusanya@jefferson.edu
(O.T. Okusanya)

Pneumomediastinum

Jordan Grewal, MD[a], Erin Alexis Gillaspie, MD, MPH[b],*

KEYWORDS

- Pneumomediastinum • Esopahgeal perforation • Boerhaave syndrome • Macklin phenomenon

KEY POINTS

- Pneumomediastinum has a wide variety of causes.
- Iatrogenic causes are a frequent etiology of pneumomediastinum.
- Workup should be focused on ruling out causes requiring urgent intervention and those that can result in significant morbidity and mortality.
- Computed tomographic scan and fluoroscopy are effective in evaluating the esophagus and defining pathology.

INTRODUCTION

Pneumomediastinum, defined as air within the mediastinal space, is the manifestation of a wide array of physiologic, interventional, and disease processes. This article reviews the epidemiology, etiology, and pathophysiology of pneumomediastinum as an independent pathologic and physiologic entity, as well as reviews the workup and management of those patients who are diagnosed with pneumomediastinum.

ANATOMY

The mediastinum, bounded by the lungs and defined by the mediastinal pleural folds, is subdivided into anterior, superior, middle, and posterior compartments defined both by anatomic landmarks and the structures within each compartment. The superior mediastinum is bordered by the thoracic outlet superiorly, the transverse thoracic plane, medial border of the pleural sacs, and the dorsal surface of the sternum. The anterior compartment is sometimes combined with the superior mediastinum and is bounded by the pericardium, pleural sacs, the sternum, and the costal cartilages. These 2 spaces contain the thymus, pericardial fat, and may contain structures such as the parathyroid glands, lymphatic tissue, and portions of the thyroid.[1] The middle compartment is formed from the pericardial sac anteriorly and posteriorly, the medial borders of the pleura laterally, and the diaphragm inferiorly. It is also known as the visceral mediastinum because it contains the viscera of the chest—the heart, trachea, esophagus, great vessels of the heart, and neural structures.[1] The posterior compartment of the mediastinum is bordered by the middle compartment anteriorly, the costophrenic angle laterally, and thoracic vertebrae posteriorly. It does not contain any thoracic viscera but does contain the sympathetic chain.[1,2]

EPIDEMIOLOGY

The overall reported incidence of pneumomediastinum (combined spontaneous and secondary) varies widely, ranging from 1 in 7000 to 45000.[3,4] Studies performed in the blunt trauma population have found that 2.2% to 4.7% of patients imaged following blunt mechanisms have radiologic evidence of pneumomediastinum[5–7]; however, this may be as high as 10% in patients with severe blunt thoracic or cervical trauma. Between 5% and 10% of these patients may have clinically significant mediastinal organ injury.[3] There is a distinct male predominance in both spontaneous and secondary pneumomediastinum and most patients are younger than 40 years.[3,5–18]

Mortality has never been reported as a consequence of spontaneous pneumomediastinum,

[a] Department of General Surgery, Vanderbilt University Medical Center, Nashville TN, USA; [b] Department of Thoracic Surgery, Creighton University Medical Center, Omaha, NE, USA
* Corresponding author. 7500 Mercy Road, Omaha, NE 68124
E-mail address: ErinGillaspie@Creighton.edu

Thorac Surg Clin 34 (2024) 309–319
https://doi.org/10.1016/j.thorsurg.2024.06.001
1547-4127/24/© 2024 Elsevier Inc. All rights reserved, including those for text and data mining, AI training, and similar technologies.

and recurrence is low, reported as 0% to 4.5%.[18] However, there can be significant morbidity and mortality associated with secondary pneumomediastinum, generally accounting for the type or severity of underlying injury.[5,7,11] Factors associated with worse outcome include air in the posterior mediastinum, air in all compartments of the mediastinum, and concomitant pleural effusion or hemothorax.[5]

CLASSIFICATION AND ETIOLOGY

Pneumomediastinum is generally separated into 2 major categories—spontaneous and secondary (**Fig. 1**). Spontaneous pneumomediastinum is defined as pneumomediastinum not the result of trauma, ingestion, or iatrogenic intervention. Secondary pneumomediastinum is any air within the mediastinum that develops as a sequela of some clear underlying pathology or injury.

Spontaneous pneumomediastinum is considered a diagnosis of exclusion, and therefore, care must be taken to rule out all secondary causes in the initial workup. Risk factors for spontaneous pneumomediastinum include a history of asthma or Chronic obstructive pulmonary disease (COPD) smoking, and drug use.[3,12,16] Common causes of spontaneous pneumomediastinum include asthma attacks or coughing fits, childbirth (prolonged Valsalva), repeated bouts of vomiting (without esophageal perforation), and rarely, inhalational drug use.

Secondary pneumomediastinum can be classified further into iatrogenic, traumatic, and nontraumatic categories. Instrumentation is the most common cause of pneumomediastinum generally resulting from tracheobronchial and esophageal injury and may include endoscopy, ultrasonography (transesophageal echo as an example), or the placement of tubes.[3] Other iatrogenic causes of pneumomediastinum include ventilator barotrauma, and, rarely, medication toxicity.[10]

Traumatic causes of pneumomediastinum are broadly classified as either blunt or penetrating. Blunt esophageal injury is rare and typically requires a high-speed mechanism.[3] More commonly, pneumomediastinum is associated with either blunt or penetrating chest wall injury to the ribs or sternum resulting in underlying injury to the lungs or airway.

Additional, secondary causes include Boerhaave syndrome or caustic ingestion with resultant esophageal injury, rupture, and pneumomediastinum. Infectious etiologies associated with pneumomediastinum include dental infections with descending mediastinitis (Ludwig's angina), acute mediastinitis, retroperitoneal infections from gasproducing organisms, and pulmonary cavitary infections.[19]

Finally, as a special case, we must consider severe acute respiratory syndrome and COVID-19, which have both been associated with pneumomediastinum. Pneumomediastinum was recognized as a distinct complication of infection with early viral variants with some studies reporting prevalence in as many as 25% of patients.[20] The incidence was notably higher in patients requiring mechanical ventilation and was proposed to be secondary to a phenomenon called the Macklin effect.[21]

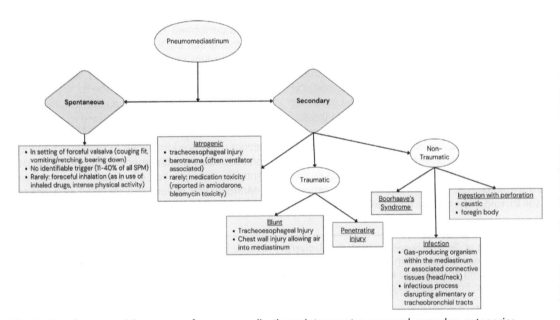

Fig. 1. Flowchart organizing causes of pneumomediastinum into spontaneous and secondary categories.

PATHOPHYSIOLOGY AND MECHANISM OF INJURY
Spontaneous/Primary Pneumomediastinum

Spontaneous pneumomediastinum is air within the mediastinum with no obvious underlying etiology (ie, no history of trauma, procedure, etc.). The mechanism underlying spontaneous pneumomediastinum was first described and experimentally proven by Macklin and Macklin in 1944 and is now known as the Macklin effect.[22] Using a cat model, Macklin and Macklin found that the pressure gradient between the intra-alveolar space and the interstitial space results in the rupture of peripheral alveoli, with air movement from the alveolus into the interstitial space, then the connective tissue sheaths of the pulmonary vasculature. This air continues along the path of least resistance—the anatomic planes of the bronchovascular bundles—making its way centrally to the hilum of the lung, and into the mediastinum (**Figs. 2** and **3**).

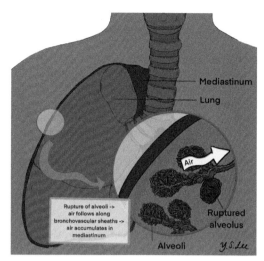

Fig. 3. Pathophysiology of spontaneous pneumomediastinum. (Image courtesy of Yeonsoo Sara Lee, MD.)

This Macklin effect accounts for more than 95% of cases of pneumomediastinum including in patients with asthma exacerbations, positive pressure ventilation in the setting of underlying pulmonary injury, and even blunt chest trauma.[23]

Described causes of spontaneous pneumomediastinum include smoking, vigorous athletic activities, cough related to Valsalva, snorting, labor, sneezing, severe retching and vomiting, and sex.[3,12,16]

Secondary Pneumomediastinum

Chest wall injury and lung injury
Traumatic injury to the sternum or anterior ribs overlying the mediastinum can create a tract through which air can travel through the soft tissues and into the mediastinum during the inspiratory phase when the intrathoracic pressure decreases, creating a negative pressure gradient.

Injury may also result in alveolar parenchymal injury that can manifest as pneumothorax, subcutaneous emphysema, or pneumomediastinum. The distribution of air within the mediastinum is useful in diagnosis and localizes to sites of injury.

Tracheobronchial injury
Tracheobronchial injury is a rare cause of pneumomediastinum.[23] The mechanism of injury may be blunt trauma, although the majority of these will cause death at the time of injury or on transport to the hospital. Penetrating trauma and iatrogenic traumas (intubation) account for the majority of tracheobronchial injuries. Index of suspicion must be high for timely identification and management.[19,24]

Other less common etiologies of tracheobronchial disruption include direct invasion of a tumor,

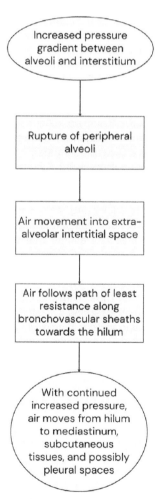

Fig. 2. The Macklin effect: flowchart detailing the mechanism of spontaneous pneumomediastinum.

implanted hardware or even granulomatous, and cavitation pulmonary infections.[19]

Esophageal injury

Esophageal injury resulting in rupture or perforation can occur due to several causes, all of which are potentially deadly. The 2019 World Journal of Emergency Surgery (WJES) consensus guidelines divide esophageal injury into 4 major categories—foreign body ingestion, caustic ingestion, esophageal perforation (both iatrogenic and spontaneous), and esophageal trauma. Each may manifest with pneumomediastinum as a result of full-thickness disruption of the esophagus.[25]

Ingestion of a caustic substance—whether alkaline or acidic—may result in necrosis of the esophageal wall and can progress to perforation. Esophageal perforation as noted earlier may be the result of spontaneous cause such as Boerhaave syndrome that is the rupture of the esophagus secondary to severe straining most commonly in the setting of repeated forceful vomiting. More commonly, an esophageal perforation results from iatrogenic causes—that is, endoscopy. Rarely, ingestion of a foreign body such as button batteries, fish bones, toothpicks, or other objects can cause esophageal perforation and pneumomediastinum.[25]

Esophageal trauma is rare, accounting for only 15% of all esophageal injuries, and is estimated to affect less than 1% of patients with trauma. The mechanism can be sharp, blunt, or, rarely, due to barotrauma from blast injuries. Isolated traumatic esophageal injuries are rare, and the typical presentation is in a polytrauma patient with injuries of the surrounding structures. Penetrating injuries are far more likely to cause pneumomediastinum than blunt injury.[25]

Iatrogenic pneumomediastinum: non-esophageal

Iatrogenic causes of pneumomediastinum not related to aerodigestive injury include dental or otolaryngologic (ENT) procedures, abdominopelvic procedures with insufflation or iatrogenic injury to a hollow viscus within the abdomen. In dental procedures, the most common culprit is the use of tools that emit compressed air, which can inadvertently enter the submandibular space via the subcutaneous tissue surrounding the surgical incision and subsequently dissect through cervical fascial planes. Once air extends to the pharyngeal and retropharyngeal planes, it can progress toward the mediastinum.[26] In otolaryngology (ENT) procedures, extensive dissection in the fascial planes of the neck, specifically the pretracheal fascial plane and the visceral space of the neck, can inadvertently introduce air, and as this space invests the trachea and esophagus, air can descend this plane into the mediastinum.[19]

Abdominopelvic procedures using insufflation or hollow organ injuries have in rare circumstances presented with pneumomediastinum.[27] There are 2 proposed etiologies: intraperitoneal air moves through the diaphragmatic hiatus alongside the esophagus into the thorax or in the retroperitoneum tracks up the retroperitoneal space into the chest.[19,28] The former is likely the source of mediastinal air after abdominopelvic insufflation. Injury to hollow viscera such as the stomach, small bowel or colon may result in intraperitoneal or retroperitoneal air as the colon and small bowel each have retroperitoneal components.

Workup

Pneumomediastinum is rare and can present as the manifestation of a benign, self-limited condition or a complication of an underlying disease-carrying high morbidity and mortality. Spontaneous pneumomediastinum is significantly more common than injury to the esophagus or the trachea; however, the signs and symptoms overlap significantly with those of Boerhaave syndrome among other secondary etiologies. Therefore, a high index of suspicion must be maintained, and further investigation must be appropriately undertaken to rule out these life-threatening conditions.

Evaluation and management should be dictated by history and clinical presentation. Multiple algorithms have been proposed[17,29]; ours is adapted from established algorithms weaving in current guidelines for the workup of esophageal and tracheobronchial injury (**Fig. 4**).

Initial workup begins with a thorough history and physical examination. Patients with spontaneous pneumomediastinum often describe a triggering event—commonly severe coughing fits, asthma, retching, or an activity involving a forceful Valsalva.[3,7–10,12–18,29] Those with secondary pneumomediastinum may describe a history of forceful, repetitive vomiting and chest pain, recent iatrogenic manipulation of the aerodigestive tract, or with a history of some other inciting event such as an ingestion event, recent surgery, or trauma.[3,5–7,11,16]

Patients describe a variety of presenting symptoms including most commonly chest pain (11%–100%), dyspnea (18%–88%%), and cough (4%–77%). Less common symptoms include neck and chest swelling, cervical pain, dysphagia, odynophagia, dysphonia, and abdominal pain. Case reports describe anxiety as the only presenting symptom; however, it is unclear whether this is a manifestation of the pneumomediastinum or other injury with subclinical presentation and

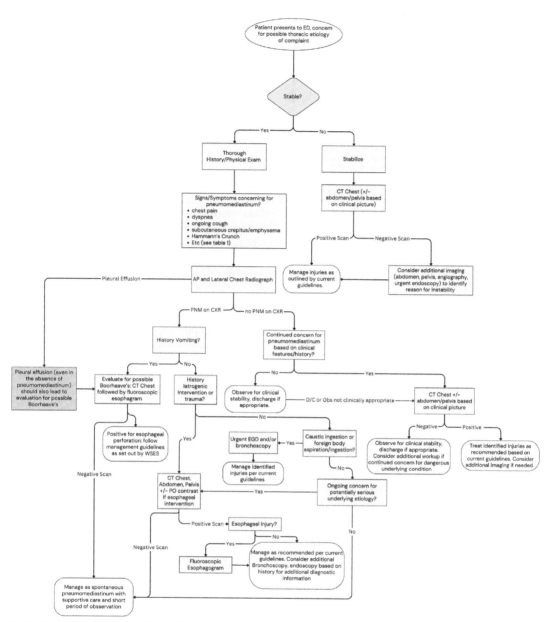

Fig. 4. Algorithm for the workup of pneumomediastinum for the workup of a patient presenting with signs or symptoms concerning for pneumomediastinum.

tachycardia.[3,5–18,29,30] In 10% of cases, there were no symptoms and pneumomediastinum is found incidentally (**Table 1**).

Physical examination is often unrevealing; however, some cases are notable for crepitus over the neck or chest, tachypnea, or Hamman's sign (rasping or crunching sound synchronous with each systole heard over the pericardium). Despite being considered pathognomonic for pneumomediastinum, it is identified in fewer than 50% of patients with confirmed pneumomediastinum on imaging.[9,12–14,17,29,30] Subcutaneous emphysema

or crepitus along the chest, neck or shoulders, and face (less commonly) can be identified in up to 83% of patients.[3,5–18,29,30]

Definitive diagnosis of pneumomediastinum requires imaging. Chest radiograph is diagnostic in 61% to 100% of patients with spontaneous or nontraumatic pneumomediastinum (11%–47% of traumatic pneumomediastinum) and should be the first step in evaluating a patient with mechanism suggestive of chest or mediastinal injury and symptoms worrisome for mediastinal pathology. Further all chest radiographs should be assessed for the

Table 1
Presenting signs and symptoms of pneumomediastinum

Symptoms		
	Chest Pain	10%–100%
	Dyspnea	18.3%–88.3%
	Cough	3.7%–77%
	Neck pain	2.4%–55.6%
	Dysphagia	8.0%–27%
	Odynophagia	6.1%–26.5%
	Abdominal pain	11%–23.5%
	Anxiety	0%–22%
	Altered mental status	4.7%–13.4%
Signs		
	Subcutaneous emphysema	2.5%–83.3%
	Rhinolalia (nasal voice quality)	22.7%–66%
	Hammans sign	5.6%–40.9%
	Neck swelling	6%–22.7%
	Hoarseness	2.4%–6%
Objective Data		
	Elevated WBC count	30%–66%
	Fever	3%–22%

presence of air regardless of presenting symptoms. Radiographic signs of pneumomediastinum include a pleural line with lucency around the mediastinal structures, a well-defined lucency surrounding the right pulmonary artery (known as the "ring around the artery" sign), air surrounding the aorta and its major branches (the "tubular aorta" sign), a continuous left diaphragm with separating the inferior border of the heart from the diaphragm, and/or air outlining the descending aorta, extending laterally between the parietal pleura land the left hemidiaphragm (the Naclerio V sign). Of note, in some patients, anterior mediastinal air may be the only finding, and identification requires a lateral film.[31,32]

Air-fluid levels, pleural effusion, and/or pneumothorax should increase suspicion for secondary pneumomediastinum requiring further workup or intervention. A pleural effusion should increase the index of suspicion for esophageal, while pneumothorax is a strong negative predictor of esophageal injury but should raise flags for possible lung or tracheobronchial injury.[3]

Additional studies are not required in most cases of pneumomediastinum and should be obtained only in an appropriate clinical context.[5]

In the setting of diagnostic uncertainty, further workup of pneumomediastinum can include computed tomographic (CT) scans, fluoroscopy, and endoscopy. Due to its ready availability, CT scan is most commonly performed (**Fig. 5**). In a patient clinically stable enough to tolerate further imaging, a CT scan can help characterize the etiology of a pneumomediastinum and distinguish location and severity of injury.

CT scan findings suggesting a spontaneous etiology of pneumomediastinum include small air lucencies surrounding bronchovascular bundles and peripheral pulmonary interstitium (at the hilum), both of which are signs of alveolar rupture.[23] This is also called the double bronchial wall sign. Other findings of pneumomediastinum include a CT ring around the artery sign, where air is seen encircling the pulmonary artery.[33]

In patients with tracheobronchial injury, CT findings include disruption of the tracheal or bronchial rings, irregularity or thickening of the membranous trachea, and massive pneumomediastinum.

Esophageal injury may manifest with esophageal wall thickening, extravasation of esophageal contents into the chest, contained fluid collections adjacent to the esophagus, and in some cases, the direct site of injury or perforation may be identified.[32,34] Detection of esophageal perforations with CT is improved when both oral and intravenous contrast are used.[35]

Fluoroscopic esophagram is also valuable in the diagnosis and characterization of esophageal perforation and should be considered in a patient with a history, physical, or other imaging concerning for possible esophageal perforation.[8] In patients with esophageal injury, contrast leak out of the esophagus is diagnostic of perforation[36]; however, the sensitivity is slightly less than a CT scan with a miss rate of 10% to 12% for barium and 22% to 50% with water-soluble contrast. Therefore, a confirmatory study is recommended for a negative esophagram. A negative water-soluble study can be followed with barium or either by a CT scan.[16,35,36] Care should be taken not to administer Gastrografin (water-soluble contrast) to patients at risk for aspiration to reduce the risk of Gastrografin-induced pneumonitis. Because an esophagram cannot rule out tracheobronchial injuries, we recommend CT and esophagogram in conjunction to evaluate patients with suspected aerodigestive injury.

Point of care ultrasound (POCUS) has been reported as being used to diagnose pneumomediastinum with some rapidity in the emergency department; however, there are no data examining its overall utility. Findings in POCUS indicative of a pneumomediastinum are the "air-gap sign" that represents accumulating air obscuring normal cardiac structures, and artifact or a-lines with loss of the parasternal and apical views, preserving the subxiphoid view (this finding differentiates between pneumomediastinum and pneumopericardium).[4]

Bronchoscopy and esophagogastroduodenoscopy (EGD) individually or in combination are

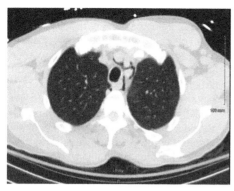 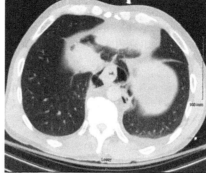

Fig. 5. Pneumomediastinum on CT scan secondary to esophageal perforation superior mediastinum (*left*) and middle inferior mediastinum (*right*).

also used to assist in diagnosis and management of pneumomediastinum.

An esophageal injury may occur secondary to an endoscopic procedure in which case further evaluation and concomitant treatment with stenting can be performed same procedure. EGD may also be used to evaluate a patient with caustic or foreign body injection to evaluate the extent and location of injury. Caution should be maintained as insufflation or manipulation of a partial thickness injury may result in full thickness injury. Visible disruption of the wall is considered diagnostic.

Bronchoscopy is the gold standard for detecting tracheobronchial injury and should be performed even in the absence of clear finding on CT if there is a high index of suspicion for tracheobronchial injury—such as suspicious traumatic mechanism, large pneumothorax and pneumomediastinum, and tension pneumomediastinum. Flexible bronchoscopy and rigid bronchoscopy are both diagnostically and therapeutically useful options.[37]

Management

The management of pneumomediastinum is dependent on the etiology and we will review the most common in the following section.

Spontaneous

Often considered benign or incidental, the management of spontaneous pneumomediastinum requires that secondary etiologies be definitively ruled out either via careful history and physical examination, imaging or endoscopic or procedural exploration. Treatment is aimed at symptoms only.[38] Many patients are admitted for 24 h inpatient observation to ensure stability and no development of signs/symptoms concerning for a missed underlying aerodigestive injury. Clinical stability, tolerating a diet intake, and improvement of symptoms are criteria for safe discharge.[39] In

studies exploring the hospitalization needs of patients with spontaneous pneumomediastinum, symptoms were universally self-limited and lasted only a few days.[29]

Rarely, patients with spontaneous pneumomediastinum may develop tension physiology, either due to associated pneumothorax or their existing pneumomediastinum. These patients should be treated with decompression via tube thoracostomy or thoracotomy/video assisted thoracoscopic surgery (VATS) mediastinal decompression on a case-by-case basis. Further management includes appropriate postoperative VATS/thoracotomy pain management, tube removal when air leak resolves and drainage is appropriately low. Furthermore, these patients should be evaluated for underlying injuries as progression to tension physiology in spontaneous pneumomediastinum is rare.[39]

Esophageal perforation

The management of esophageal perforation as outlined by the WJES falls under 3 categories: nonoperative, endoscopic, and surgical. Nonoperative management that generally consists of nil per os, intravenous (IV) hydration, and antibiotics to cover aerobes, anaerobes, and fungal organisms should be initiated in all patients with suspicion for esophageal perforation while workup is underway. Patients who are clinically stable and in whom the perforation is contained may be managed expectantly with careful monitoring and availability of specialized services in the event of progressive symptoms. A follow-up esophagogram 3 to 7 days after the initial presentation is used to assess for improvement or resolution.[25] Up to 25% of patients can be managed in this manner, and nonoperative treatment can continue as long as the patient remains clinically stable.[40] Should the patient decline clinically, CT of the chest with IV and oral contrast is indicated to evaluate for progression of the perforation.

Nutrition is a critical consideration. If PO intake is likely to be delayed, alternate feeing considerations via enteral tube or total parenteral nutrition (TPN) should be initiated. The use of endoscopically guided or image-guided feeding tube placement is preferred over blind placement.

Transmural perforation, mediastinal contamination, and pleural contamination require procedural intervention. Management of the perforation may be approached endoscopically with the use of clips, endostitch, stenting, and endoscopic vacuum therapy. Endoscopic intervention has been the gold standard for injuries that occur and are recognized during an endoscopic procedure and has become the first choice for many institutions for most esophageal perforations regardless of etiology.[25] Clips can be used on defects of varying sizes and can be done either through or over the scope. Endostitch is less commonly used but gaining popularity and is useful as it can be successfully used to close edematous, friable tissue not as amenable to clips. However, these techniques require a level of technical skill that may not be available in all centers. Stenting is the most commonly utilized endoscopic treatment method and is safe and effective even in the case of mediastinal contamination. It has an esophageal salvage rate of up to 80%.[25,40] Stents remain in place for 2 to 4 weeks. Benefits of stenting include complete exclusion of the esophageal injury; such that oral enteral nutrition can be resumed much more quickly compared to other methods. Endoscopic vacuum therapy is a newer technique in which a wound vacuum device is used within the lumen of the damaged esophagus over the injury. It can be used to avoid damage control surgery and reduce morbidity and mortality. These techniques are often coupled with a pleural and mediastinal washout via transthoracic approach with wide drainage.

Surgical intervention is indicated in all patients who do not meet nonoperative criteria, who fail stenting and washout or who present late with significant contamination, or significant destruction of the esophagus either due to mechanism or injury or malignancy. Intervention should be initiated promptly in parallel with resuscitative efforts as delay greatly increases morbidity and mortality of esophageal perforations.

Surgical approach and laterality are determined by the location of the injury—left-sided cervical approach for the upper esophagus, a right-sided transthoracic for mid-esophagus, left-sided transthoracic for distal esophagus, and trans-abdominal for gastroesophageal junction (GEJ) with suspected intra-abdominal contamination.[25,40] Surgical options include washout of the pleura and the mediastinum, debridement of the esophagus and either stenting or primary repair, esophageal diversion, or even esophagectomy. Primary repair is preferred, when possible, as it preserves native anatomy and eliminates the need for further reconstructive operations. Principles of primary repair include myotomy to expose the entire mucosal defect, closure of the mucosal, muscularis propria, consideration of soft tissue coverage, and a contralateral myotomy. A malignant perforation, large (>10 cm) defect, and diffuse necrosis preclude the ability to perform primary repair. Esophageal diversion is preferred in patients who have large perforations with extensive thoracic contamination, with malignant perforation, or end-stage achalasia. While esophagectomy is always a consideration, most patients are not sufficiently stable and diversion with control of infection, time for recovery and resuscitation is critical to good outcome. Staged reconstruction can occur once a patient has completely recovered. If a patient is too unstable or unhealthy to undergo even a diversion, a T-tube can be placed to create a controlled fistula for diversion, with distal enteral feeding access.[25,40]

Tracheal injury

Management of a patient in whom there is a concern for tracheobronchial injury always begins with assuring adequacy of airway and breathing. Negative pressure is ideal to avoid extension of pneumomediastinum. However, some patients may require intubation with positioning of the endotracheal tube distal to the site of injury. Once the airway is secured and the full extent of the injury has been assessed via imaging and bronchoscopy, management can proceed.

Treatment is based on the size of the injury and the extent of associated damage. The most common pattern of iatrogenic injury is a membranous tear extending down the right mainstem airway. Penetrating traumatic injuries are highly variable in both position and size. Thoughtful resuscitation should be undertaken. The role of empiric antibiotics is debated.[39]

In patients who do not require supplemental oxygen to maintain adequate saturation, injuries up to 4 cm with minimal contamination can be treated conservatively, with supportive treatment and regular endoscopic follow-up until the injury is completely healed. Even patients requiring intubation for respiratory support can be managed successful with an endotracheal tube (ETT) positioned distal to the injury. Contemporary literature supports the conservative management of larger injuries.

Stenting across the defect, the use of fibrin glue, and other endobronchial repair techniques are also gaining popularity and are a safe intervention for smaller injuries and in patients who are unable to tolerate surgical intervention[37]

Tracheal or bronchial membranous injuries that are full thickness with broad communication to the mediastinum and large air leak and complex injuries involving other mediastinal organs or injury with significant contamination will typically require an operative approach to repair.

Approach to a proximal tracheal injury is accomplished via cervical incision, whereas the distal trachea and proximal mainstem are via right transthoracic approach. In an emergency setting, a right thoracotomy is used more commonly than minimally invasive or VATS approach. A sternotomy may be used if there are concomitant cardiac injuries; however, some portions of the airway are more difficult to reach from an anterior approach.

Repair technique varies from simple primary closure with absorbable sutures for a laceration. Resection and reconstruction with end-to-end anastomosis may be required for a more complex injury. Pedicled intercostal flaps can be used to buttress the repair.[37–51] Extensive destruction of the trachea may require reconstruction with vascularized flaps to replace portions of the tracheal or bronchial wall. Ideally a patient should be extubated and returned to negative pressure ventilation as soon as possible after repair; however, if additional sites of injury prohibit extubating, a tube should be left distal to the repair.

Concomitant airway and esophageal injuries should be attempted to be primarily repaired and importantly must include the interposition of soft tissue—a pericardial or intercostal flap—to prevent future development of tracheoesophageal fistula.[37]

SUMMARY

Pneumomediastinum is defined as air within the mediastinum. While for many patients, this is a benign finding with no clear underlying cause; in some cases, this may be indicative of an esophageal or tracheal injury that is accompanied by high morbidity and mortality. A high index of suspicion coupled with history, physical, laboratory, and radiographic testing must carefully rule out secondary causes requiring intervention. Iatrogenic instrumentation is the most common cause of both esophageal and tracheal injury resulting in pneumomediastinum, and blunt trauma is the most common traumatic cause of pneumomediastinum. Spontaneous pneumomediastinum requires only supportive treatment, while aerodigestive injury requires additional workup for localization and evaluation, and intervention.

CLINICS CARE POINTS

- Pneumomediastinum, defined as air in the mediastinum, is often a benign finding without clinical consequence.
- Iatrogenic instrumentation is the most common cause of tracheal and esophageal injury.
- Blunt injury is the most common cause of traumatic pneumomediastinum.
- A comprehensive history and physical combined with diagnostic studies such as imaging can help to determine potential cause and morbidity.
- Ruling out underlying esophageal, tracheal or underlying cause requiring intervention is critical.

DISCLOSURE

J. Grewal and E. Gillaspie - no pertinent dislocues. Consults for Astra Zeneca, BMS, Genentech and Intuitive Surgical. Speaker for BMS and Intuitive Surgical.

REFERENCES

1. Agarwal PP. The ring-around-the-artery sign. Radiology 2006;241(3):943–4.
2. Al-Mufarrej F, Badar J, Gharagozloo F, et al. Spontaneous pneumomediastinum: diagnostic and therapeutic interventions. J Cardiothorac Surg 2008;3:59.
3. Aslaner MA, Kasap GN, Demir C, et al. Occurrence of pneumomediastinum due to dental procedures. Am J Emerg Med 2015;33(1):125.e1–3.
4. Aujayeb A. Patient centered care for spontaneous pneumomediastinum: a step in the right direction. J Thorac Dis 2023;15(3):964–6.
5. Banki F, Estrera AL, Harrison RG, et al. Pneumomediastinum: etiology and a guide to diagnosis and treatment. Am J Surg 2013;206(6):1001–6. ; discussion 1006.
6. Bejvan SM, Godwin JD. Pneumomediastinum: old signs and new signs. AJR Am J Roentgenol 1996;166(5):1041–8.
7. Brand M, Bizos DB, Burnell L. A review of non-obstetric spontaneous pneumomediastinum and subcutaneous emphysema. S Afr J Surg 2011;49(3):135–6.
8. Lentz RJ, Floyd JE. Mediastinitis and fibrosing mediastinitis. In: Broaddus VC, Schnapp LM, Stapleton RD, et al, editors. Murray and Nade's textbook of respiratory medicine. 7th edition. Philadephia, PA: Elsevier; 2022. p. 1605–17.

9. Caceres M, Ali SZ, Braud R, et al. Spontaneous pneumomediastinum: a comparative study and review of the literature. Ann Thorac Surg 2008;86(3): 962–6.

10. Caceres M, Braud RL, Maekawa R, et al. Secondary pneumomediastinum: a retrospective comparative analysis. Lung 2009;187(5):341–6.

11. Chan MSM, Chan IYF, Fung KH, et al. High-resolution CT findings in patients with severe acute respiratory syndrome: a pattern-based approach. AJR Am J Roentgenol 2004;182(1):49–56.

12. Chao D. Air, air everywhere. Am Fam Physician 2003;68(7):1381–3.

13. Chapdelaine J, Beaunoyer M, Daigneault P, et al. Spontaneous pneumomediastinum: are we over investigating? J Pediatr Surg 2004;39(5):681–4.

14. Chassagnon G, Favelle O, Derogis V, et al. Spontaneous pneumomediastinum due to the macklin effect: less is more. Intern Emerg Med 2015;10(6): 759–61.

15. Chawla A. Imaging in noncardiovascular thoracic emergencies: a pictorial review. Singapore Med J 2015;56(11):604–10. quiz 611.

16. Chen YH, Lin PC, Chen YL, et al. Point-of-care ultrasonography helped to rapidly detect pneumomediastinum in a vomiting female. Medicina (Kaunas) 2023;59(2):394.

17. Chirica M, Kelly MD, Siboni S, et al. Esophageal emergencies: WSES guidelines. World J Emerg Surg 2019; 14(1):26.

18. Cristina D, Damarco F. Upper airways tract in emergency settings. In: Bissacco D, Settembrini AM, Mazzari A, editors. Primary management in general, vascular and thoracic surgery. Switzerland: Springer International Publishing; 2022. p. 49–62.

19. Dionísio P, Martins L, Moreira S, et al. Spontaneous pneumomediastinum: experience in 18 patients during the last 12 years. J Bras Pneumol 2017;43(2): 101–5.

20. Dwarakanath A, Horgan L, Jayawardena M, et al. The clinical course of pneumomediastinum in patients with SARS-CoV-2 before invasive mechanical ventilation. Clin Med 2022;22(3):271–5.

21. Ferguson M. Mediastinum. In: Ferguson M, editor. Thoracic surgery Atlas. Philadelphia, PA: Elsevier; 2024. p. 150–73.

22. Gerazounis M, Athanassiadi K, Kalantzi N, et al. Spontaneous pneumomediastinum: a rare benign entity. J Thorac Cardiovasc Surg 2003;126(3):774–6.

23. Hülsemann P, Vollmann D, Kulenkampff D. Spontaneous pneumomediastinum-hamman syndrome. Dtsch Arztebl Int 2023;120(31–32):525.

24. Almansa C, Achem SR. Non-cardiac chest pain of non-esophageal origin. In: Kaski JC, Eslick GD, Bairey Merz CN, editors. Chest pain with normal coronary arteries: a multidisciplinary approach. London: Springer; 2013. p. 9–21.

25. Khaitan PG, Famiglietti A, Watson TJ. the etiology, diagnosis, and management of esophageal perforation. J Gastrointest Surg 2022;26(12):2606–15.

26. Kouritas VK, Papagiannopoulos K, Lazaridis G, et al. Pneumomediastinum. J Thorac Dis 2015;7(Suppl 1): S44–9, 01.11.

27. Kourounis G, Lim QX, Rashid T, et al. A rare case of simultaneous pneumoperitoneum and pneumomediastinum with a review of the literature. Ann R Coll Surg Engl 2017;99(8):e241–3.

28. Lee WS, Chong VE, Victorino GP. Computed tomographic findings and mortality in patients with pneumomediastinum from blunt trauma. JAMA Surg 2015; 150(8):757–62.

29. Macklin MT, Macklin CC. Malignant interstitial emphysema of the lungs and mediastinum as an important occult complication in many respiratory diseases and other conditions: an interpretation of the clinical literature in the light of laboratory experiment. Medicine 1944;23(4):281–358.

30. MacLeod JBA, Tibbs BM, Freiberger DJ, et al. Pneumomediastinum in the injured patient: inconsequential or predictive? Am Surg 2009;75(5):375–7.

31. Maunder RJ, Pierson DJ, Hudson LD. Subcutaneous and mediastinal emphysema. pathophysiology, diagnosis, and management. Arch Intern Med 1984; 144(7):1447–53.

32. Molena D, Burr N, Zucchiatti A, et al. The incidence and clinical significance of pneumomediastinum found on computed tomography scan in blunt trauma patients. Am Surg 2009;75(11):1081–3.

33. Molina G, Contreras R, Coombes K, et al. Pneumomediastinum as a complication of cocaine insufflation. Cureus 2023;15(5):e38392.

34. Mondello B, Pavia R, Ruggeri P, et al. Spontaneous pneumomediastinum: experience in 18 adult patients. Lung 2007;185(1):9–14.

35. Morgan CT, Kanne JP, Lewis EE, et al. One hundred cases of primary spontaneous pneumomediastinum: leukocytosis is common, pleural effusions and age over 40 are rare. J Thorac Dis 2023;15(3): 1155–62.

36. Neupane R, Lam W, Marks JM. Esophageal perforation. In: Docimo S, Pauli EM, editors. Clinical algorithms in general surgery. Switzerland: Springer International Publishing; 2019. p. 139–41.

37. Newcomb AE, Clarke CP. Spontaneous pneumomediastinum: a benign curiosity or a significant problem? Chest 2005;128(5):3298–302.

38. Overcast WB, Taylor C, Capps AE, et al. Utility of fluoroscopic oesophagography in the setting of spontaneous and blunt traumatic pneumomediastinum. Clin Radiol 2023;78(3):e214–20.

39. Özdemir S, Bilgi DÖ, Hergünsel GO, et al. Incidence and risk factors for pneumomediastinum in COVID-19 patients in the intensive care unit. Interact Cardiovasc Thorac Surg 2022;34(2):236–44.

40. Parkar N, Javidan-Najad C, Bhalla S. The mediastinum, including the pericardium. In: Grainger and Allison's diagnostic radiology. 7th edition. Philadelphia, PA: Elsevier; 2021. p. 67–103.
41. Sahni S, Verma S, Grullon J, et al. Spontaneous pneumomediastinum: time for consensus. N Am J Med Sci 2013;5(8):460–4.
42. Takada K, Matsumoto S, Hiramatsu T, et al. Management of spontaneous pneumomediastinum based on clinical experience of 25 cases. Respir Med 2008;102(9):1329–34.
43. Townsend CM, editor. Sabiston textbook of surgery: the biological basis of modern surgical practice. 21st edition. Philadelphia, PA: Elsevier; 2022.
44. Van Deusen MA, Crye M, Levy J. Esophageal injury. In: Rodriguez A, Barraco RD, Ivatury RR, editors. Geriatric trauma and acute care surgery. Swizterland: Springer International Publishing; 2018. p. 167–72.
45. Wei CJ, Levenson RB, Lee KS. Diagnostic utility of CT and fluoroscopic esophagography for suspected esophageal perforation in the emergency department. AJR Am J Roentgenol 2020;215(3):631–8.
46. Welter S, Essaleh W. Management of tracheobronchial injuries. J Thorac Dis 2020;12(10):6143–51.
47. Wintermark M, Schnyder P. The macklin effect. Chest 2001;120(2):543–7.
48. Yang S, Chiu T, Lin T, et al. Subcutaneous emphysema and pneumomediastinum secondary to dental extraction: a case report and literature review. Kaohsiung J Med Sci 2006;22(12):641–5.
49. Yu MH, Kim JK, Kim T, et al. Primary spontaneous pneumomediastinum: 237 cases in a single-center experience over a 10-year period and assessment of factors related with recurrence. PLoS One 2023;18(7):e0289225.
50. Yudin A. Ring around artery sign, double bronchial wall sign. In: Metaphorical signs in computed tomography of chest and abdomen. Springer International Publishing; 2023. p. 83.
51. Alemu B, Yeheyis ET, Tirineh AG. Spontaneous primary pneumomediastinum: is it always benign? J Med Case Rep 2021;15:157.

What Is New with Cervical Perforations? A Clinical Review Article

Hope Conrad, MD, Praveen Sridhar, MD*

KEYWORDS

- Cervical esophageal perforations • Esophageal disease • Endoscopic techniques
- Endovac therapy

KEY POINTS

- Cervical esophageal perforations are usually iatrogenic in nature, occurring most frequently as a result of endoscopic instrumentation.
- After prompt diagnosis, appropriate initial treatment of cervical esophageal perforations includes initiation of nil-per-os status and administration of broad-spectrum antibiotics, intravenous fluids, and nutrition via enteral access.
- Small defects without signs of systemic disease may be managed conservatively.
- Large defects, perforations with traumatic etiology, and/or presence of hemodynamic instability warrant operative intervention.
- Based on limited studies, novel endoscopic techniques offer promising methods of minimally invasive intervention for the management of esophageal perforations.

BACKGROUND

Esophageal perforations are historically uncommon but are associated with poor outcomes. While most esophageal perforations are iatrogenic in nature, less frequent etiologies include Boerhaave's syndrome, malignancy, trauma, and toxic ingestion.[1] Survival associated with esophageal perforation has significantly improved overtime, with mortality rates down trending from 18% to 10% over the last 25 years.[2] Despite this improvement, mortality from this disease remains relatively high. Prompt diagnosis and treatment have been associated with improved outcomes, as have improvements in perioperative management.[3,4]

Perforations most frequently occur within the thoracic esophagus, followed by the cervical and abdominal esophagus.[4,5] Unlike thoracic perforations, the management of cervical esophageal perforations is highly variable.[6,7] Clinical decision-making can be nuanced and often requires consideration of individual clinical scenario. Appreciation of cervical esophageal anatomy is imperative to understanding disease progression as well as deciding on method of intervention. A wide range of interventions are currently available to treat cervical perforations, including nonoperative, endoscopic, and operative management options.

DISCUSSION
Anatomy of the Cervical Esophagus

The cervical esophagus extends from the lower border of the cricoid cartilage to the level of the sternal notch. Coursing posterior to the trachea and anterior to the spinal column, the cervical esophagus is anchored to the prevertebral fascia along C6–T2. At this level, the muscular layer of the

Division of Thoracic Surgery, Department of Surgery, University of Arizona, 1625 North Campbell Avenue, Tucson, AZ, USA
* Corresponding author. 1501 North Campbell Avenue, Room #4302, P.O. Box 245071, Tucson, AZ 85724.
E-mail address: psridhar@arizona.edu

Thorac Surg Clin 34 (2024) 321–329
https://doi.org/10.1016/j.thorsurg.2024.05.005
1547-4127/24/© 2024 Elsevier Inc. All rights are reserved, including those for text and data mining, AI training, and similar technologies.

cervical esophagus is thin and there is no serosal layer to provide additional support, increasing risk of perforation.[6,8] The physiologic narrowing caused by the cricopharyngeal and inferior constrictor muscles also increases risk of perforation, and most iatrogenic esophageal perforations occur at this location.[1,6] Fortunately, because of adherence to prevertebral fascial planes, cervical perforations are often self-contained.[4] The outcomes of cervical esophageal perforations are less severe than those of thoracic and abdominal perforations, with a mortality of 6% compared to 10.9% and 13.2%, respectively.[9,10] This is likely due to limited spread of contamination, allowing for local drainage and avoidance of a thoracotomy or laparotomy.[4] Because of its proximity to the anterior cervical spine, the cervical esophagus is also at risk for iatrogenic perforations due to spinal surgery from orthopedic hardware as well as spontaneous rupture secondary to osteophytes.[4]

Diagnosis and Initial Management

The diagnostic pathway for cervical esophageal perforations is similar to that of thoracic and abdominal perforations. The first step in evaluation is a detailed history and physical examination. Common findings associated with esophageal perforations include pain, odynophagia, subcutaneous emphysema, and hemodynamic instability.[3] Findings specific to cervical perforations may include dysphagia, dysphonia, pain induced with neck flexion, and erythema, edema, or induration of the soft tissues of the neck.[4,11,12] Any of these signs and symptoms, particularly in the setting of recent instrumentation or existing esophageal disease, should prompt high suspicion of esophageal perforation. A timely diagnosis is imperative to maximizing patient outcomes and survival.[3]

The study typically used in the initial diagnosis of esophageal perforation is an upper gastrointestinal swallow study with water-soluble contrast. When positive, this study demonstrates location of the perforation and extent of disease. However, water-soluble contrast carries a high false-negative rate, especially in the upper esophagus.[4,12,13] Swallow studies using barium contrast have higher specificity and can be used in the setting of negative findings and high clinical suspicion.[4,12] Barium contrast is not used in the initial diagnosis due to risk of mediastinitis.[14] Another method of diagnostic imaging includes an oral-contrasted computed tomographic (CT) esophagram. While this has not historically been recommended as initial imaging for diagnosis of esophageal perforation, this technique is widely available and can be performed without the need of a fluoroscopy team.[3] Additionally, there is

mounting evidence that CT esophagram can be more sensitive than fluoroscopic examination.[4]

Because most cervical esophageal perforations occur from endoscopy, some cases may be diagnosed at the time of injury.[4] However, the use of endoscopy to diagnose esophageal perforations is controversial. Endoscopy in the setting of esophageal perforation is associated with risk of full-thickness conversion of partial-thickness defects and tension pneumothorax formation from insufflation. Endoscopy does provide the ability to directly visualize and characterize the injury and viability of the surrounding tissue. This technique also provides the option of immediate therapeutic intervention. The use of endoscopy is often reserved for cases of critically ill and/or intubated patients who are unable to participate safely in radiological studies as well as cases with high clinical suspicion despite negative imaging.[3]

Treatment Options

The management of cervical esophageal perforation is less well-studied than perforations in other regions of the esophagus. Consequently, there is no single best practice recommendation for treatment.[4] Regardless of management strategy, all patients diagnosed with esophageal perforation should be made nil-per-os (npo) and started on broad-spectrum antibiotics, enteral nutrition, and intravenous fluid resuscitation.[3] Further treatment course is dependent on patient clinical status and disease. Patients found to have small defects while demonstrating hemodynamic stability may be treated with nonoperative management. Perforations associated with hemodynamic instability, large mucosal defects, widespread contamination, as well as those with delayed presentation or diagnosis warrant surgical intervention[6] (**Table 1**). While novel endoscopic procedures are being studied in the management of cervical perforations, there are limited data on the efficacy of these interventions. There have been smaller studies, case series, and case reports of successful management using endoscopic stents, clips, sutures, negative pressure therapy, and adhesives (**Table 2**).

Nonoperative management

Patients who are hemodynamically stable with a defect smaller than 1 cm may initially be managed medically if no signs of free extravasation are seen on imaging.[6,12] Nonoperative management includes hospital admission, strict npo status, broad-spectrum antibiotic initiation, and nutrition via enteric or parenteral access.[6] If the patient remains stable, a repeat swallow study should be obtained in 5 to 7 days to reassess the perforation prior to allowing oral intake.[7,12] Clinical deterioration during

Table 1
Operative, nonoperative, and combined technique interventions

Author	Study Design	# Of Cervical Perforations	Etiology of Perforation[a]	Intervention	Outcomes
Tang et al,[15] 2021	Retrospective	18/335 patients	Mixed	• 17 patients with primary repair • 1 patient with diversion	• Cervical perforations more likely to have repair ($P = .0001$)
Abbas et al,[51] 2009	Retrospective	26/119 patients	Mixed	• 15 operative • 11 nonoperative	• Cervical perforations with 8% mortality compared to 14% overall
Aghajanzadeh et al,[16] 2015	Retrospective	26/26 patients	Mixed	• Primary repair: 38.46% • Primary repair and drainage: 26.92% • Drainage alone: 19.23% • Stenting: 11.53% • Esophagectomy and J tube 15.4%	• Overall mortality: 7.7% • High mortality among esophagectomies • 21.4% of patients who had drainage as part of their treatment experienced drain leaks
Bhatia et al,[17] 2011	Retrospective	15/119 patients	Mixed	• 10 primary repair • 1 palliative care • 2 drainage • 1 resection	• 7.6% mortality among patients with perforations in cervical esophagus
Bufkin et al,[18] 1996	Retrospective	9/66 patients	Mixed	• 5 operative • 4 nonoperative	• No mortalities for nonoperative management
Eroglu et al,[19] 2009	Retrospective	14/44 patients	Mixed	• 11 primary repair • 3 nonoperative	• No mortalities • 2 leaks in operative group
Schmidt et al,[20] 2010	Retrospective	8/62 patients	Mixed	• 6 primary repair • 2 nonoperative	• No mortality in cervical perforation group
Montminy et al,[21] 2023	Retrospective	8/32 patients	Iatrogenic	• 3 endoscopic (2 self expanding metal stent [SEMS], 1 clips) • 4 nonoperative • 1 operative	• 25% mortality • Both within upper esophageal sphincter (UES), both endoscopic ultrasound (EUS) related
Sarr et al,[13] 1982	Retrospective	18/47 patients	Iatrogenic	• 3 nonoperative • 15 operative repair (3 primary repair + drainage, 12 drainage only)	• 1 death in nonoperative group • 0 death in operative group • 1 patient in nonoperative group required later drainage • 4 patients in the operative group developed fistulas and 1 developed abscess

[a] Etiology describes the cause of perforation, including iatrogenic, spontaneous, traumatic, caustic, foreign body related, and malignant. Mixed etiology describes studies with 2 or more etiologies included within the sample size.

Table 2
Endoscopic interventions

Authors	Study Design	# Of Cervical Perforations	Etiology of Perforation[a]	Intervention	Outcomes
Bae,[22] 2019	Case study	1 patient[b]	Spontaneous	Injection of glue	• Resolved
Parapar Alvarez et al,[23] 2023	Retrospective	1 patient	Spontaneous	Endovac therapy	• Resolved • Treatment duration: <3 wk • 4 endovac changes
Loeck et al,[24] 2021	Retrospective	5/10 patients	Iatrogenic	Endovac therapy	• 100% rate of closure • Treatment duration median: 7.6 d • Average of 2 changes per treatment
Kimura et al,[25] 2013	Case study	1 patient	Foreign body	Injection of fibrin glue	• Resolved
Takahashi et al,[26] 2017	Retrospective	1/17 patients	Iatrogenic	Endoscopic clip placement	• Resolved
Freeman et al,[27] 2012	Retrospective	15/187 patients	Mixed	Endoscopic stent	• 4/15 cervical perforation patients failed stent therapy • Cervical perforation has higher rates of stent failure compared to thoracic
Yoon et al,[28] 2015	Case report	1 patient	Foreign body	Endovac therapy	• Resolved
Fischer et al,[29] 2007	Case series	1/4 patients	Malignant	Endoscopic clip placement	• Resolved
Gerke et al,[30] 2007	Case report	1 patient	Iatrogenic	Endoscopic clip placement	• Resolved
Jung et al,[31] 2021	Retrospective analysis	1/7 patients	Iatrogenic	Endovac therapy	• Successful treatment • 12 endovac changes
Kumbhari et al,[32] 2015	Case series	2 patients	Iatrogenic	Fully covered self-expanding metallic stents	• Resolved within 3 d • Had to remain intubated during therapy
Horvath et al,[33] 2018	Retrospective	7/43 patients	Mixed	3 diagnostic endoscopy and medical management, 4 therapeutic endoscopy[c]	• No mortality
Ben-David et al,[34] 2014	Retrospective	2 patients	Iatrogenic	Removable covered stent placement	• Resolved
Anoldo et al,[35] 2017	Case report	1 patient	Iatrogenic	10 d of drainage followed by glue injection	• Resolved
Wasano et al,[36] 2014	Case Report	1 patient	Iatrogenic	Endoscopic suturing using laparoscopic needle driver and knot pusher	• Resolved

[a] Etiology describes the cause of perforation, including iatrogenic, spontaneous, traumatic, caustic, foreign body related, and malignant. Mixed etiology describes studies with 2 or more etiologies included within the sample size.
[b] Patient initially diagnosed with perforation, but prolonged treatment ultimately led to fistula at time of glue.
[c] Therapeutic endoscopy describes interventions using stents, clips, endovacs, or drains.

this period of observation should prompt reimaging and surgical exploration.

Initial conservative management of cervical esophageal perforations has been found to have better success rates compared to thoracic perforations, with a 13% failure rate compared to 62%.[4] One study demonstrated that npo status between injury and diagnosis affects outcomes, as patients who remain npo fare better with conservative measurement.[7]

Mechanism of perforation has also been found to affect outcomes. Though most cases of cervical perforation are iatrogenic in nature, approximately 15% are secondary to penetrating trauma.[15] Several studies have reported improved outcomes associated with early surgical intervention in cases of traumatic cervical esophageal perforation.[7] Thus, it may be prudent to pursue operative intervention in the setting of trauma even if the patients appear stable or have small defects.

Endoscopic management

Significant advances in the field of endoscopy over the years have expanded interventions available to gastroenterologists and surgeons. There are limited data regarding endoscopic management of cervical esophageal perforations relative to intrathoracic perforations.

Esophageal stent placement is the most frequently utilized intervention in cases of intrathoracic esophageal perforation, but stenting in the cervical esophagus is considered relatively contraindicated due to the risk of airway compression and compromise, migration, and patient discomfort.[3,16] However, this technique has been implemented successfully in the literature.[15,17–19] Most perforations are categorized by region rather than by specific measurement, and there are no recommendations on cervical stent placement based on level of perforation. Stenting of proximal cervical perforations spanning the hypopharynx has been described, but patients required intubation to mitigate risk of airway compromise. In these cases, patients remained in the intensive care unit until stents were removed on post-procedure day 3.[19] In contrast, intrathoracic stent management generally occurs over the course of several weeks prior to replacement over removal.[20]

Endoscopic clipping has been successfully used to treat esophageal perforations with success rates of 59% to 83%.[21] Through-the-scope clipping is recommended for defects less than 1 cm, while over-the-scope clipping is recommended for defects 1 to 2 cm.[22] There is no need for clip removal, precluding the need for further intervention after successful treatment.[23] Endoscopic clipping within the cervical esophagus has been described in case

studies with successful resolution of perforation.[24–27] An alternative method of primary closure is endoscopic suturing (**Fig. 1**).[6,28] Wasano and colleagues describe endoscopic suture closure of an iatrogenic esophageal injury spanning the pharynx and hypopharynx using a laparoscopic needle holder and knot pusher with complete resolution of the injury.[28] Because these techniques do not offer source control in cases of contamination, they are limited to patients with small defects, good tissue quality, and limited contamination of the cervical soft tissues.[22]

Endoscopic vacuum therapy (EVT), or endovac therapy, is a relatively new technique in the management of esophageal perforations. This intervention is performed by placing a sponge at the tip of a nasogastric tube within the perforation bed and applying negative pressure therapy. This system reduces bacterial contamination while promoting wound healing.[22] The sponge can be placed over the luminal defect or within the cavity itself, allowing for drainage of contamination while facilitating wound closure.[29] The use of EVT is not well described in the cervical esophagus compared to other regions, but successful case reports have been reported in the literature.[29–32] Drawbacks to this therapy include patient discomfort and need for repetitive procedures for sponge change. This therapy can also be limited by proximity to carotid sheath due to bleeding risk.[20,32]

The use of adhesives has been described for the treatment of various esophageal perforations. These include cyanoacrylate glue plugs, polyglycolic acid sheet sealant, and fibrin glue. These measures have been described more frequently for iatrogenic perforations of the middle and lower esophagus, but implementation in the cervical esophagus perforations has only been described in case reports.[24,33–36]

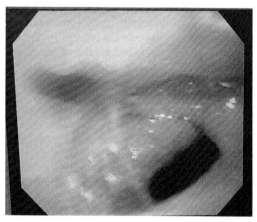

Fig. 1. Cervical esophageal perforation on esophagogastroduodenoscopy (EGD).

Surgical management

Surgical management of cervical esophageal perforations is always warranted in patients with instability, delayed presentation, and significant contamination. Principally, the management of the contaminated space is no different from any other, and the most straightforward intervention is open surgical drainage alone via cervicotomy through the left neck.[6] Perforations that occur in the cervical esophagus are often contained within the prevertebral space, allowing for open operative drainage without extensive dissection and collateral damage to surrounding structures. This has been associated with lower rates of morbidity compared to open drainage of thoracic and abdominal disease, which require access through thoracotomy or laparotomy.[4]

Following opening of the prevertebral space, accurate assessment of the perforation and viability of the surrounding tissue is mandatory. Whenever possible, primary repair should be performed following adequate debridement of nonviable esophageal tissue.[3] The full extent of mucosal injury should be exposed by opening the muscular layers longitudinally cephalad and caudal to the mucosal perforation.[12,37] If primary repair is not feasible secondary to the quality of tissue or the size of the defect, debridement and drainage can be followed by T-tube placement. This technique creates a controlled esophago-cutaneous fistula that can be managed overtime with T-tube removal when the patient's contamination is controlled and nutritional status improves.[14] T-tube placement is typically reserved for critically ill patients, allowing for timely source control.[38]

When primary repair is possible, it is performed by drainage and thorough debridement of the area followed with 2 layer closure. Longitudinal myotomy is again sometimes required to visualize the full extent of the mucosal defect to allow for a complete mucosal repair.[3] Primary repair can be augmented with muscle flap creation for additional reinforcement with vascularized tissue. Addition of a flap has been found to reduce risk of sepsis and accelerate initiation of feeding. Because the cervical esophagus is vulnerable to injuries related to cervical spine hardware or osteophytes, flaps also serve to provide a layer of protection in the prevertebral space.[6] Options for flaps include rotated sternocleidomastoid muscle (SCM), omohyoid, or strap muscles due to their proximity.[4] SCM flaps have demonstrated lower morbidity than other flaps, but patients may develop chronic neck pain or functional deficits secondary to spinal accessory nerve injury.[39] For small perforations, omohyoid flaps may be more appropriate as they are associated with decreased risk of pain.[6,7]

Perforations in the cervical esophagus are often contained, making them amenable to localized drainage. However, in critically ill patients or in cases primary repair cannot be achieved, esophageal diversion can be performed.[14] Diversion in esophageal perforation has a mortality of 23%, much higher than 11% reported in patients who undergo primary repair. However, diversion has been found to have improved outcomes in patients who are critically ill.[40] When performing a diversion, an end esophagostomy is created and externalized through the left neck. While creation of a side esophagostomy has been described, it is not frequently performed due to technical difficulty, habitus limitations, and risk of incomplete diversion.[41,42] After diversion, the remaining esophagus is reduced into the abdomen and the hiatal diaphragm is closed.[2,14] Alternatively, esophageal exclusion is a technique in which the esophagus is stapled distal to the perforation and left in place to heal.[3] Patients can pursue reconstruction 6 to 12 months after diversion.[2,3,14]

Esophageal diversion and exclusion leave the gastrointestinal tract in discontinuity, requiring enteric access for nutrition and decompression. This can be achieved by placement of a gastrostomy or gastrojejunostomy tube. These adjuncts may also be warranted in cases that require prolonged npo status while the space is being decontaminated, as enteral nutrition is preferable to parenteral.[6]

Looking to the Future

The outcomes of esophageal perforations have improved overtime, likely secondary to improvement in perioperative management, diagnostic technology, and surgical technique.[2,43] Management trends have also changed with a decreased rate of surgical diversion and increased rate of primary repair from 2005 to 2020.[2] While there are limited studies describing the effect of endoscopic interventions on esophageal perforation outcomes, development of new technology has certainly broadened the armamentarium of treatment options available to interventionalists. Endoscopic therapy has gained traction to the point that it is now well established in the algorithm for management of intrathoracic perforations. As these data accumulate and stent technology improves, this may translate to increased use in the cervical esophagus. Similarly, endovac therapy is now becoming a frequently employed method of managing intrathoracic perforations and anastomotic leaks following esophagectomy. It may be considerably more tolerable than stents within the cervical esophagus in critically ill patients and may accelerate closure of defects when combined with drainage of the prevertebral space.

The literature is limited with regard to endoscopic management of cervical perforation at this time. In addition to techniques that have been applied to intrathoracic perforations, there are even more novel and innovative endoscopic techniques do show promise in the treatment of cervical esophageal perforations. For example, the combination of endovac and stent placement, aptly described as the sponge-over-stent technique, has been described in small studies in upper gastrointestinal perforations.[20] While it has been used for postoperative leaks in the cervical esophagus, it has yet to be determined whether this can be applied to patients with cervical perforations.[44,45] Cellular therapies may also yield some advancements in the future as authors have described the injection of emulsified adipose tissue stromal vascular fracture into esophageal fistulas resulting in successful closure of cervical esophageal fistulas.[46] While the need has moved relatively slowly in the arena of cervical perforations, these opportunities offer the possibility of continued progress in patient outcomes after cervical esophageal perforation.[47–50]

SUMMARY

The outcome of esophageal perforations is influenced by time to diagnosis/treatment, location and extent of the perforation, etiology of injury, and patient comorbidities. Unlike other regions of the esophagus, determining best treatment of cervical esophageal perforations is controversial and nuanced. All esophageal perforations warrant hospital admission for monitoring, initiation of broad-spectrum antibiotics, implementation of strict npo status, and provision of early nutrition via enteral or parenteral access. Further management with conservative, endoscopic, or operative measures is chosen based on individual patient factors. In the case of critically ill patients, operative intervention is always warranted to achieve prompt source control. Otherwise, some patients may be appropriately treated with medical or endoscopic management. While conservative and operative management has remained relatively unchanged in the management of cervical esophageal perforations, innovations in endoscopic technology have broadened the treatment options available to this patient population. Endoscopic stents, clips, sutures, endovac therapy, and adhesives have been described in the successful management of cervical esophageal perforations, but continued research is necessary to understand best application of these techniques within this patient population.

CLINICS CARE POINTS

- Prompt diagnosis and initiation of treatment is associated with improved esophageal perforation outcomes.
- Initial management includes admission for careful monitoring and implementation of broad-spectrum antibiotic coverage, nutrition via enteral or parenteral access, intravenous fluid resuscitation, and strict npo status.
- Conservative management can be successful in carefully selected patients without evidence of systematic disease, while hemodynamic instability always warrants prompt surgical intervention.
- Endoscopic techniques have been successfully used to treat cervical esophageal perforations, providing a minimally invasive procedural intervention.
- Endoscopic clips, sutures, and adhesives allow for primary repair.
- Endovac therapy and stent placement provide methods of source control while the defect heals secondarily.
- More research is needed to understand the population of patients who would benefit most from endoscopic intervention.

DISCLOSURE

There are no commercial or financial conflicts of interest nor are there any funding sources associated with the authors.

REFERENCES

1. Brinster CJ, Singhal S, Lee L, et al. Evolving options in the management of esophageal perforation. Ann Thorac Surg 2004;77(4):1475–83.
2. Wong LY, Leipzig M, Liou DZ, et al. Surgical Management of Esophageal Perforation: Examining Trends in a Multi-Institutional Cohort. J Gastrointest Surg 2023;27(9):1757–65.
3. Khaitan PG, Famiglietti A, Watson TJ. The Etiology, Diagnosis, and Management of Esophageal Perforation. J Gastrointest Surg 2022;26(12):2606–15.
4. Chen S, Shapira-Galitz Y, Garber D, et al. Management of Iatrogenic Cervical Esophageal Perforations: A Narrative Review. JAMA Otolaryngol Head Neck Surg 2020;146(5):488–94.
5. Sdralis E, Ilias K, Petousis S, et al. Epidemiology, diagnosis, and management of esophageal perforations: systematic review. Dis Esophagus 2017;30(8):1–6.

6. Bourhis T, Mortuaire G, Rysman B, et al. Assessment and treatment of hypopharyngeal and cervical esophagus injury: Literature review. Eur Ann Otorhinolaryngol Head Neck Dis 2020;137(6):489–92.

7. Zenga J, Kreisel D, Kushnir VM, et al. Management of cervical esophageal and hypopharyngeal perforations. American Journal of Otolaryngology - Head and Neck Medicine and Surgery 2015;36(5):678–85.

8. Akgoz Karaosmanoglu A, Ozgen B. Anatomy of the Pharynx and Cervical Esophagus. Neuroimaging Clin N Am 2022;32(4):791–807.

9. Biancari F, D'Andrea V, Paone R, et al. Current treatment and outcome of esophageal perforations in adults: Systematic review and meta-analysis of 75 studies. World J Surg 2013;37(5):1051–9.

10. Navarro R, Javahery R, Eismont F, et al. The Role of the Sternocleidomastoid Muscle Flap for Esophageal Fistula Repair in Anterior Cervical Spine Surgery. Spine (Phila Pa 1976) 2005;30(20):E617–22.

11. Fairbairn K, Worrell SG. Esophageal Perforation: Is Surgery Still Necessary? Thorac Surg Clin 2023;33(2):117–23.

12. Nirula R. Esophageal Perforation. Surgical Clinics of North America 2014;94(1):35–41.

13. Sarr M, Pemberton J, Payne WS. Management of instrumental perforations of the esophagus. J Thorac Cardiovasc Surg 1982;84:211–8.

14. Lampridis S, Mitsos S, Hayward M, et al. The insidious presentation and challenging management of esophageal perforation following diagnostic and therapeutic interventions. J Thorac Dis 2020;12(5):2724–34.

15. Tang A, Ahmad U, Raja S, et al. Repair, Reconstruct, or Divert Fate of the Perforated Esophagus. Ann Surg 2021;274(5):E417–24.

16. Aghajanzadeh M, Porkar NF, Ebrahimi H. Cervical Esophageal Perforation: A 10-Year Clinical Experience in North of Iran. Indian J Otolaryngol Head Neck Surg 2014;67(1):34–9.

17. Bhatia P, Fortin D, Inculet RI, et al. Current concepts in the management of esophageal perforations: A twenty-seven year Canadian experience. Ann Thorac Surg 2011;92(1):209–15.

18. Bufkin BL, Miller JI, Mansour KA. Esophageal Perforation: Emphasis on Management.; 1996.

19. Eroglu A, Turkyilmaz A, Aydin Y, et al. Current management of esophageal perforation: 20 years experience. Dis Esophagus 2009;22(4):374–80.

20. Schmidt SC, Strauch S, Rösch T, et al. Management of esophageal perforations. Surg Endosc 2010;24(11):2809–13.

21. Montminy EM, Jones B, Heller JC, et al. Endoscopic iatrogenic esophageal perforation and management: a retrospective outcome analysis in the modern era. BMC Gastroenterol 2023;23(1). https://doi.org/10.1186/s12876-023-03004-x.

22. Bae SH. Transcatheter embolization of the esophagomediastinal fistula with N-butyl cyanoacrylate glue: A case report. Int J Surg Case Rep 2019;65:73–7.

23. Parapar Álvarez L, Cerrella Cano C, Andrés Vargas González C, et al. Endoscopic endoluminal therapy with the Eso-SPONGE® system for the treatment of spontaneous esophageal perforation with associated paraoesophageal collection. Rev Esp Enferm Dig 2023;115(10):589.

24. Loeck J, von Lücken HJ, Münscher A, et al. Endoscopic negative pressure therapy (ENPT) in head and neck surgery: first experiences in treatment of postoperative salivary fistulas and cervical esophageal perforations. Eur Arch Oto-Rhino-Laryngol 2021;278(11):4525–34.

25. Kimura T, Takemoto T, Fujiwara Y, et al. Esophageal perforation caused by a fish bone treated with surgically indwelling drainage and fibrin glue injection for fistula formation. Ann Thorac Cardiovasc Surg 2013;19(4):289–92.

26. Takahashi R, Yoshio T, Horiuchi Y, et al. Endoscopic tissue shielding for esophageal perforation caused by endoscopic resection. Clin J Gastroenterol 2017;10(3):214–9.

27. Freeman RK, Ascioti AJ, Giannini T, et al. Analysis of unsuccessful esophageal stent placements for esophageal perforation, fistula, or anastomotic leak. Ann Thorac Surg 2012;94(3):959–65.

28. Yoon BW, Yi KI, Kang JH, et al. Negative pressure wound therapy for cervical esophageal perforation with abscess. Auris Nasus Larynx 2015;42(3):254–7.

29. Fischer A, Schrag HJ, Goos M, et al. Nonoperative treatment of four esophageal perforations with hemostatic clips. Dis Esophagus 2007;20(5):444–8.

30. Gerke H, Crowe GC, Iannettoni MD. Endoscopic Closure of Cervical Esophageal Perforation Caused By Traumatic Insertion of a Mucosectomy Cap. Ann Thorac Surg 2007;84(1):296–8.

31. Jung CFM, Müller-Dornieden A, Gaedcke J, et al. Impact of Endoscopic Vacuum Therapy with Low Negative Pressure for Esophageal Perforations and Postoperative Anastomotic Esophageal Leaks. Digestion 2021;102(3):469–79.

32. Kumbhari V, Azola AA, Tieu AH, et al. Iatrogenic pharyngoesophageal perforations treated with fully covered self-expandable metallic stents (with video). Surg Endosc 2015;29(4):987–91.

33. Horvath P, Lange J, Stüker D, et al. Multimodal Treatment Strategies for Esophageal Perforation, Available at: www.surgical-laparoscopy.com, Accessed February 12, 2024. 2018.

34. Ben-David K, Behrns K, Hochwald S, et al. Esophageal perforation management using a multidisciplinary minimally invasive treatment algorithm. J Am Coll Surg 2014;218(4):768–74.

35. Anoldo P, Manigrasso M, Milone F, et al. Case report of a conservative management of cervical esophageal

perforation with acrylic glue injection. Annals of Medicine and Surgery 2018;31:11–3.

36. Wasano K, Hashiguchi S, Suzuki N, et al. Transoral closure of pharyngeal perforation caused by gastrointestinal endoscopy. Auris Nasus Larynx 2014; 41(1):113–7.

37. Chirica M, Champault A, Dray X, et al. Esophageal perforations. J Vis Surg 2010;147(3). https://doi.org/10.1016/j.jviscsurg.2010.08.003.

38. Binda C, Jung CFM, Fabbri S, et al. Endoscopic Management of Postoperative Esophageal and Upper GI Defects—A Narrative Review. Medicina (Lithuania) 2023;59(1). https://doi.org/10.3390/medicina59010136.

39. Takeshita N, Ho KY. Endoscopic closure for full-thickness gastrointestinal defects: Available applications and emerging innovations. Clin Endosc 2016;49(5):438–43.

40. Paspatis GA, Dumonceau JM, Barthet M, et al. Diagnosis and management of iatrogenic endoscopic perforations: European Society of Gastrointestinal Endoscopy (ESGE) Position Statement. Endoscopy 2014;46(8):693–711.

41. Gurwara S, Clayton S. Esophageal Perforations: An Endoscopic Approach to Management. Curr Gastroenterol Rep 2019;21(11). https://doi.org/10.1007/s11894-019-0730-5.

42. Kasuga K, Hosaka H, Sato K, et al. Endoscopic tissue shielding with polyglycolic acid sheet, fibrin glue, and endoclip for perforation during balloon dilation for esophageal stricture after endoscopic submucosal dissection. Clin J Gastroenterol 2022; 15(2):320–4.

43. Seehawong U, Morita Y, Nakano Y, et al. Successful treatment of an esophageal perforation that occurred during endoscopic submucosal dissection for esophageal cancer using polyglycolic acid sheets and fibrin glue. Clin J Gastroenterol 2019;12(1): 29–33.

44. Hanwright PJ, Purnell CA, Dumanian GA. Flap reconstruction for esophageal perforation complicating anterior cervical spinal fusion: An 18-year experience. Plast Reconstr Surg Glob Open 2015;3(5). https://doi.org/10.1097/GOX.0000000000000350.

45. Treffalls JA, Jacobsen CP, Das NA, et al. Delayed Esophageal Reconstruction: Indications, Techniques, and Outcomes. Foregut. The Journal of the American Foregut Society 2023. https://doi.org/10.1177/26345161231212388.

46. Raymond DP, Watson TJ. Esophageal Diversion. Operat Tech Thorac Cardiovasc Surg 2008;13(2): 138–46.

47. Deng Y, Hou L, Qin D, et al. Current treatment and outcome of esophageal perforation: A single-center experience and a pooled analysis. Medicine (United States) 2021;100(16):E25600.

48. Valli PV, Mertens JC, Kröger A, et al. Stent-over-sponge (SOS): A novel technique complementing endosponge therapy for foregut leaks and perforations. Endoscopy 2018;50(2):148–53.

49. Lange J, Dormann A, Bulian DR, et al. VACStent: Combining the benefits of endoscopic vacuum therapy and covered stents for upper gastrointestinal tract leakage. Endosc Int Open 2021;09(06):E971–6.

50. Nachira D, Trivisonno A, Costamagna G, et al. Successful Therapy of Esophageal Fistulas by Endoscopic Injection of Emulsified Adipose Tissue Stromal Vascular Fraction. Gastroenterology 2021; 160(4):1026–8.

51. Abbas G, Schuchert MJ, Pettiford BL, et al. Contemporaneous management of esophageal perforation. Surgery 2009;146(4):749–55.

Endoscopic Management of Iatrogenic Perforations

Sarah Clifford, BS, Corey Kelsom, PharmD, MS, Evan T. Alicuben, MD*

KEYWORDS

- Esophageal perforation • Stent • Clip • Endoscopic vacuum therapy

KEY POINTS

- Endoscopic management of iatrogenic esophageal perforations is a viable strategy for stable patients without significant mediastinal or peritoneal contamination.
- Stent placement is the most widely used endoscopic strategy, with an 85% to 90% clinical success rate.
- Fixing a stent by clip or suture helps prevent stent migration.
- Clip placement, vacuum therapy, and suturing are possible leak closure strategies requiring advanced endoscopic skills.

INTRODUCTION

Esophageal perforation continues to present a diagnostic and therapeutic challenge. The rarity of the condition and its nonspecific presentations contribute to controversy over approaches to early management and treatment. Although rare, esophageal perforation is a life-threatening condition with a mortality ranging from 10% to 29%.[1,2] Contributing to the mortality risk include the timing of the diagnosis, degree of contamination, and size of the perforation.

The rate of iatrogenic perforation of the esophagus is increasing in parallel with the rapid development and utilization of upper gastrointestinal (GI) endoscopic techniques.[1] Decades of clinical experience and innovation in surgical technique have made various treatment options available, ranging from observational medical therapy to radical esophagectomy. Notably, in optimized candidates under specific conditions, nonoperative treatment of perforations and percutaneous control of mediastinal sepsis offers an alternative to traditional management with open, primary repair.[3] Herein, the etiology and diagnostic approach to iatrogenic esophageal perforations are briefly reviewed, followed by a review of the current options for endoscopic closure.

NATURE OF THE PROBLEM
Etiology

Iatrogenic injury to the esophagus is the most frequent cause of esophageal perforation. The reported causes of iatrogenic perforation (**Box 1**) primarily revolve around endoscopic procedures but can include esophageal instrumentation and surgery on the esophagus or adjacent structures.[4] When therapeutic procedures are performed at the time of diagnostic esophageal endoscopy, the risk of perforation increases even further.

Clinical Presentation

Early diagnosis of esophageal perforation is essential for timely and appropriate treatment to minimize morbidity and mortality.[2] However, the presentation of esophageal perforation is diverse, with a range of signs and symptoms difficult to definitively differentiate from other diagnoses. Common clinical manifestations include chest pain, dysphagia, dyspnea, subcutaneous emphysema, epigastric pain, fever,

Division of Thoracic Surgery, Department of Cardiothoracic Surgery, University of Pittsburgh Medical Center, Pittsburgh, PA, USA
* Corresponding author. 5200 Centre Avenue, Suite 715, Pittsburgh, PA 15232.
E-mail address: alicubenet@upmc.edu

Thorac Surg Clin 34 (2024) 331–339
https://doi.org/10.1016/j.thorsurg.2024.07.001
1547-4127/24/© 2024 Elsevier Inc. All rights are reserved, including those for text and data mining, AI training, and similar technologies.

Box 1
Causes of iatrogenic esophageal perforation

Endoscopic procedures (flexible and rigid)

   Diagnostic biopsy

   Therapeutic dilation (stricture, achalasia, and malignancy)

   Endoscopic resections

   Ablative procedure (photodynamic therapy, argon plasma coagulation, and neodymium doped yttrium aluminum garnet [Nd:YAG] laser therapy)

Esophageal instrumentation

   NGT insertion

   Attempted endotracheal intubation

   Transesophageal echocardiography

   Sengstaken–Blakemore or Minnesota tube placement

Surgical procedures

   Cervical: spine surgery and thyroidectomy

   Thoracic: lung resection, mediastinoscopy, and mediastinal tumor resection

   Abdominal: hiatal hernia repair and Heller myotomy

tachycardia, and tachypnea. The presence of esophageal perforation should always be suspected, along with any combination of these signs and symptoms following instrumentation of the esophagus, until proven otherwise. The cause and location of the injury, as well as the time between perforation and diagnosis, can help determine the clinical features of esophageal perforation.[5]

Cervical: generally contained in the dense anatomy of the neck. These events tend to be less severe and more easily treated. Patients present with neck pain, cervical dysphagia, dysphonia, and subcutaneous emphysema overlying the neck.

Intrathoracic: rapidly contaminates the mediastinum and thus causes progressive sepsis. Patients present with chest pain, dysphagia, dyspnea associated with tachycardia, and hypotension due to the systemic inflammatory response.

Intra-abdominal: results in contamination of the peritoneal cavity due to being uncontained. Patients present with severe epigastric or diffuse abdominal pain. Similar to intrathoracic perforations, sepsis ensues, leading to tachycardia and shock.

Diagnosis

The diagnosis of esophageal perforation should be suspected based on clinical presentation but requires objective confirmation with either contrast-enhanced imaging or endoscopic evaluation.[4]

There is a wide array of imaging findings as follows:

1. Upright chest and abdominal radiographs
   a. Subcutaneous emphysema, pleural effusion, pneumomediastinum, and hydropneumothorax
2. Esophagography with oral contrast (**Fig. 1**)
   a. Contrast leakage from the esophagus will not only locate the perforation but determine if it is contained or freely leaking into the mediastinum, pleural spaces, neck, or abdomen
3. Computed tomographic (CT) scan with oral contrast (**Fig. 2**)
   a. Extraluminal air in the soft tissues of the mediastinum, perceptible communication of the esophagus with a contiguous air–fluid collection
4. Esophagogastroduodenoscopy (EGD)
   a. Allows direct visualization of the entire esophagus and stomach to characterize the extent of injury

A patient with suspected esophageal perforation should rarely be taken for intervention without more advanced imaging. Findings from studies with oral/enteric contrast help to determine whether a perforation is contained versus extravasating into a body cavity. The extent of cavity contamination can be elucidated and, in the case of intrathoracic perforation, can dictate which pleural space should be explored. These findings can also help predict which patients a nonoperative strategy may be feasible.

INITIAL MANAGEMENT AND TREATMENT

The critical determinants of therapy for esophageal perforation are the cause, location, and severity of the perforation and the interval between perforation and treatment. Operative interventions include primary repair or esophagectomy with or without diversion with a combination of reinforcement and drainage techniques. Nonoperative strategies include medical management, endoscopic drainage, self-expandable stents, clips, suture repair, and endoscopic vacuum therapy (E-Vac). In general, this approach is utilized for limited perforations without florid sepsis. Iatrogenic perforations are uniquely situated for this strategy, given their propensity for quick diagnosis and fasting before interventions, leading to less contamination.

Irrespective of the approach, the initial management includes a nil per os status, aggressive fluid

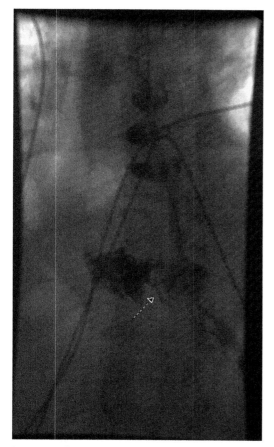

Fig. 1. Esophagram with oral contrast extravasating through defect (*arrow*).

resuscitation with hemodynamic monitoring, and broad-spectrum antibiotic coverage considering antifungal agents. Symptom control with analgesia and antiemetics is essential to prevent further injury. The patient should be watched in a closely monitored setting with serial examinations.

THERAPEUTIC OPTIONS
Esophageal Stents

Endoscopic esophageal stents restore luminal integrity to prevent further extraluminal soilage. There was a well-established role for stenting in malignant esophageal disease, which led to growing interest in benign indications such as perforation.[6] Some of the earliest reports of endoscopic management of benign perforations occurred in the late 1990s with stent placement following failed surgical repair of an esophageal leak.[7] The degree of perforation and contamination distinguishes the patients who receive stents from those who receive operative or other endoscopic interventions; however, there is limited evidence to support specific inclusion criteria.

Procedural steps

1. Position the patient supine with the arms tucked to allow for C-arm movement.
2. Perform EGD under general anesthesia to protect the airway from possible aspiration.
3. Note the level of the esophagogastric junction, the lesion's site, and the esophagus's estimated circumference. Place radio-opaque markers at the planned site of stent deployment.
4. Choose the stent based on the length of the lesion and the estimated circumference of the esophagus.
   a. Stent length should allow a minimum of 2 cm on each side of the straddled lesion. This ensures adequate coverage of the lesion and accounts for small movements of the stent with peristalsis.
   b. Larger diameter stents are often preferred as they provide optimal sealing of leaks and divert luminal contents. However, they are more likely to cause chest pain and fistula formation.

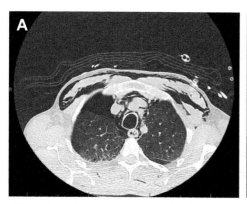
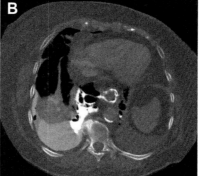

Fig. 2. CT with oral contrast demonstrates significant pneumomediastinum (*A*) and contrast extravasation into the mediastinum and right pleural space (*B*).

5. Lubricate the stent, then load on the guidewire, and pass it into the esophagus.
6. Thread the assembly over the guidewire and deploy.
7. Confirm proper positioning fluoroscopically and endoscopically (**Fig. 3**).
   a. If adjustments are needed, the stent can be grasped and moved to a more proximal point using endoscopy and fluoroscopy.
   b. If the stent is too proximal after deployment, it will likely need removal and replacement.
   c. A pneumatic esophageal dilatation balloon can expand if the stent does not open entirely after its deployment.

Clinical outcomes

In a review of available series reporting on outcomes following placement of stents for anastomotic leaks and benign esophageal perforations, Dasari and colleagues[8] found a technical success rate, defined as the ability to occlude the site of leak evidenced by the intraprocedural contrast study, of 91.4%. Technical success was more likely in patients receiving metallic than plastic stents (96.5% vs 89.8%, $P = .025$). The clinical success rate, defined as complete healing following stent placement, was 81.1% and was similar between the 2 groups. Stent migration occurred in 20.8% of patients and was more likely to occur with plastic stents. An updated systematic review published in 2020 found a similarly high technical success rate of 96% with a clinical success rate of 87%.[9] Plastic stents were associated with a significantly higher migration rate with lower technical success.

The timing of stent removal should be individualized according to the normalization of clinical, laboratory, and imaging data. It is our practice to perform stent removal and re-evaluation for the need of stent replacement approximately 3 weeks following initial placement, assuming the patient has defervesced and is ideally discharged from the hospital. It is crucial to ensure removal as increased rates of complications were realized in patients with a stent in place for more than 4 to 6 weeks.[10,11] These can be catastrophic with the formation of vascular fistulae.[12]

Stent migration and subsequent inadequate coverage of the perforation site remain a significant concern. Various endoscopic strategies have been utilized to secure stent placement. By utilizing clips, stent migration can be reduced to 10%.[13] Suturing can also be used to secure stents to prevent migration.[14,15] In a meta-analysis comparing suturing versus clips versus no intervention, suturing was associated with a significantly decreased rate of stent migration.[16] Interestingly, clips did not lead to a statistically significant lower migration rate compared to no intervention, but there was no difference between the suturing and clips groups.

Some concerns over treatment failure precluding the possibility of definitive surgical intervention may detract some providers from considering stent placement. In a study examining outcomes following stent failure for acute perforation, Ong and colleagues[17] reported a successful operative repair in 69% of patients. In 15%, an esophagectomy was required.

Endoscopic Clips

Endoscopic clipping was initially developed for the treatment of GI bleeding but has become an established treatment of esophageal perforations.[18,19] Through-the-scope (TTS) methods introduce the clip via the working channel. Instinct clip (Cook Medical, Bloomington, IN), QuickClick Pro (Olympus, Center Valley, PA), and Resolution clip (Boston Scientific, Natick, MA, USA) are the most frequently applied TTS systems. These different

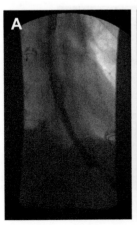
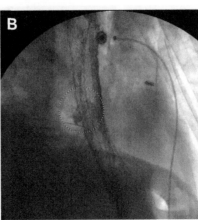

Fig. 3. Oral contrast study demonstrating adequate coverage of a perforation (*A*). Persistent contrast extravasation should prompt stent revision or alternative treatment strategy (*B*).

clips vary in rotation ability, jaw opening capacity, strength, and deployment mechanism. This approach is best utilized for perforations under 1 cm in size.

Over-the-scope (OTS) clips are loaded on a cap mounted on the endoscope's tip. Traumatic teeth on the clips are best suited for full-thickness perforations. OTS clips include the over the scope clip (OTSC) (Ovesco, Germany) and the Padlock Clip (Aponos Medical, Kingston, NH), which can suction tissue into the cap without other instrumentation. The Ovesco OTSC has a large width spanning 12 mm, designed to grasp more tissue. This approach is generally better suited for more significant defects up to 2 cm in size and friable or necrotic tissue.

Procedural steps

1. Position the patient supine under general endotracheal anesthesia or monitored sedation.
2. Perform careful diagnostic endoscopic evaluation to determine the dimensions of the perforation and location relative to the gastroesophageal (GE) junction.
3. Prepare and place the first clip in the distal portion of the tear and work proximally to avoid endoscope-induced clip displacement.
   a. TTS: Insert the clip through the working channel of the endoscope.
   b. OTS: Fit the endoscope with the cap-mounted device. Either suction the defect into the cap or grasp it with forceps before clip deployment.
4. Confirm closure with endoscopy.

Clinical outcomes

Outcomes following endoscopic clip placement for iatrogenic perforation are challenging to characterize. This approach is most commonly utilized for GI leaks; thus, most series may include esophageal perforation but as a smaller subset.[20] The overall successful closure rate ranges from 70% to 100% with a mean of 90%.[21,22] Voermans and colleagues[23] found that immediate closure was achieved in 100% of patients with esophageal perforation in a prospective multicenter cohort of acute iatrogenic GI perforations.

A review of the available series on endoscopic clip placement found that clips were most commonly used during the early diagnosis of minimally contaminated iatrogenic perforations. The success rates did not differ significantly between TTS and OTS strategies (88.8% vs 92.85%, $P > .12$).[24] The authors recommended TTS clips be used for lesions less than 10 mm in size with more extensive lesions (<20 mm) treated with OTS clips.

Endoscopic Vacuum Therapy

E-Vac uses the same treatment principles as vacuum-assisted closure therapy for external wounds.[25] Both improve and accelerate healing by removing infected secretions, reducing edema, increasing local perfusion, and promoting granulation tissue formation.[26] This therapy has most commonly been used for anastomotic leaks following esophageal or rectal resection but has also been applied to acute perforations.

The endosponge (B Braun Melsungen AG, Melsungen, Germany) is the only commercially made device for E-Vac therapy and is currently only Food and Drug Administration-approved in treating anastomotic leaks involving the rectum. The current Wound V.A.C. (Lifecell, Bridgewater, NJ) device has been adapted to perform E-Vac therapy.

Procedural steps
Primary closure

1. Position the patient supine under general endotracheal anesthesia or monitored sedation.
2. Perform careful endoscopy to determine the perforation dimensions, associated cavity, and location relative to the incisors. Irrigate and debride the cavity as much as possible.
3. Insert a nasogastric tube (NGT) through the patient's nares and retrieve it through the mouth.
4. Create an endosponge by cutting foam according to dimensions obtained during endoscopy. Create a tunnel through the long axis of the foam. Ensure that all fenestrations of the NGT will sit within the foam.
5. Suture the endosponge to the NGT by placing a permanent suture through the end of the foam and then through the tube. Secure with an air knot. Grasp the air knot with a rat tooth grasper or biopsy forceps passed through the endoscope and insert the grasped sponge into the esophagus.
6. Place the endosponge into the desired area, usually into a fistula cavity external to the esophagus. This is most effectively done by advancing the grasper into the cavity and then releasing the suture.
7. Externalize the drainage tube transnasally, fix it to the nose, and connect it to the external suction pump.

Removal

1. Interrupt the suction and disconnect the drainage tube.
2. Free the foam from the surrounding tissue by injecting 30 to 50 mL sterile water through the disconnected tube. The endosponge can also be grasped and dislodged from surrounding tissue.

3. Pull the endosponge up to the oropharynx and cut from the NGT through the mouth before removing the rest of the NGT through the nose.

Clinical outcomes

E-Vac therapy alone has been shown to close esophageal perforations with low mortality rates successfully.[27–30] Success rates of perforation closure range from 84% to 100%, with a mean of 90%.[22,28,31–34] A systematic review found successful healing in 91% is associated with an overall mortality of 12.8%.[35] Further, E-Vac therapy overcomes the physiologic negative pressure of the thorax, preventing extraluminal contamination and maintaining source control. As such E-Vac offers an endoscopic intervention to provide drainage and removal of the septic focus instead of the other endoscopic options.

A unique aspect of this management strategy is the need for relatively frequent device changes to prevent tissue ingrowth and inadequate drainage through tubing due to viscous GI secretions. Most series describe a change interval of 3 to 5 days.[26] While some authors have suggested that this may be a benefit, allowing for the opportunity to assess for healing and convert to alternative treatment strategies, there is still morbidity associated with the need for frequent changes.[36] In a recently published series, patients with acute esophageal perforation required a mean of 5 to 6 changes to achieve leak closure.[32,37,38]

Endoscopic Suture

Endoscopic suturing techniques allow defects to be pulled closed by full thickness sutures.[39]

The Overstitch device (Apollo Endosurgery, Austin, TX) consists of a handle for needle driving as well as a suture exchange catheter unit, which is attached to the control head. Sutures can be deployed and then reloaded without having to remove the endoscope.

Procedural steps

1. Place the patient in the supine position under general endotracheal anesthesia or monitored sedation.
2. Perform careful endoscopy to determine the dimensions of perforation and its location relative to the GE junction. Irrigate and debride the cavity as much as possible.
3. Insert a dual-channel therapeutic endoscope through an esophageal overtube, preloaded with the Overstitch device.
4. Place the first suture at the distal portion of the tear and work proximally with either interrupted or continuous sutures.

5. Confirm closure with endoscopy and esophagogram.

Clinical outcomes

The success of this approach is primarily limited to case reports and small series.[40] In the most extensive published series of endoscopic suturing for the management of GI defects, a success rate of 93% was found.[15] Given the full-thickness bites taken with suture, closure of edematous, friable, or necrotic tissue may be more effective than clips, which tend to grasp primarily mucosa. This approach theoretically allows for closure of more significant defects compared to clips, with some advocating for closure between 2 and 5 cm.

DISCUSSION

The evolution of complex technology has brought about the rise in the use of endoscopic approaches for what historically was an exclusively surgical diagnosis. Additionally, the availability of diagnostic modalities and vigilance from care providers performing invasive procedures can lead to earlier diagnosis of perforation, limiting contamination and increasing the likelihood of successful leak closure by endoscopic procedure alone. Nevertheless, the decision to perform endoscopic management over operative repair remains controversial, and there are no guideline-based recommendations. As opposed to other more insidious etiologies of esophageal perforation, such as chronic vomiting or cancer, the mechanism of an iatrogenic perforation can lead to a relatively limited injury site. This may lend itself to more conservative management encompassing endoscopic therapies alone.[41] However, in cases of resectable cancer, achalasia, or caustic injury, surgical management is recommended.[42]

Part of the challenge in assessing the efficacy of endoscopic options is the relatively small number of patients in case series and the heterogeneity in most case series, with very few solely examining iatrogenic esophageal perforations. Additionally, very few studies compare treatment strategies among the endoscopic options. In a series comparing 32 patients treated with E-Vac therapy with 39 patients treated with stents for anastomosis leak, E-Vac therapy was found to be an independent predictor of wound closure with a reported success rate of 84.4% compared to 53.8% for the stent group.[27]

The decision to perform stent placement versus operative repair remains controversial. In a propensity-matched analysis, Freeman and colleagues[43] found that stent placement was associated with a significant reduction in morbidity, length of stay, time to oral intake, and cost compared to operative repair. The mortality rate was similar. The decision to perform nonoperative management has been further bolstered by studies demonstrating very reliable sealing of the leak and salvage of the native esophagus.[44] Comparatively, it is associated with a significantly shorter in-hospital stay, lower risk of postoperative morbidity, and the ability to start oral liquid ingestion early.

An essential consideration for endoscopic management of iatrogenic perforations is that while this approach may avoid the morbidity of an invasive surgery, the need for reintervention is relatively high.[8,45] Nevertheless, given that the reintervention is likely via an endoscopic approach, the overall morbidity to the patient remains low. Predicting treatment failures can be difficult in a relatively rare diagnosis. In a comparative analysis, Freeman and colleagues[46] identified risk factors for stent failure following perforation, fistula, or anastomotic leak. The authors found that leak location (cervical and gastroesophageal junction) and injury length longer than 6 cm were associated with treatment failure.

SUMMARY

Iatrogenic esophageal perforations can effectively be managed via endoscopic approaches. Timely diagnosis and initial management are critical to a successful outcome. Stent placement remains the most common strategy with high rates of success. Adjunct measures to prevent migration are effective in avoiding the need for reintervention. The use of clips, suturing, and E-Vac are alternative options for perforation management, with each requiring advanced endoscopic skills. There is no clear superior option, and additional comparative studies are needed.

CLINICS CARE POINTS

- Endoscopic management of iatrogenic esophageal perforation can be considered for patients without significant contamination who are hemodynamically stable.
- Stent placement is the most widely used endoscopic strategy, with a clinical success rate of 85% to 90%.
- Use of clipping or suturing can prevent stent migration and require additional procedures.
- Metal stents are less likely to migrate than plastic stents and have a higher technical success rate.

- Clip placement, vacuum therapy, and suturing are possible strategies with success, as demonstrated in small case series.

DISCLOSURE

The authors have nothing to disclose.

REFERENCES

1. Sdralis EK, Petousis S, Rashid F, et al. Epidemiology, diagnosis, and management of esophageal perforations: systematic review. Dis Esophagus 2017;30(8).
2. Biancari F, D'Andrea V, Paone R, et al. Current treatment and outcome of esophageal perforations in adults: systematic review and meta-analysis of 75 studies. World J Surg 2013;37(5):1051–9.
3. Eroglu A, Aydin Y, Ulas AB. Minimally invasive and endoscopic approach to esophageal perforation. Eurasian J Med 2022;54(1):101–6.
4. Lampridis S, Mitsos S, Hayward M, et al. The insidious presentation and challenging management of esophageal perforation following diagnostic and therapeutic interventions. J Thorac Dis 2020;12(5):2724–34.
5. Khaitan PG, Famiglietti A, Watson TJ. The etiology, diagnosis, and management of esophageal perforation. J Gastrointest Surg 2022;26(12):2606–15.
6. Yakoub D, Fahmy R, Athanasiou T, et al. Evidence-based choice of esophageal stent for the palliative management of malignant dysphagia. World J Surg 2008;32(9):1996–2009.
7. Segalin A, Bonavina L, Lazzerini M, et al. Endoscopic management of inveterate esophageal perforations and leaks. Surg Endosc 1996;10(9):928–32.
8. Dasari BV, Neely D, Kennedy A, et al. The role of esophageal stents in the management of esophageal anastomotic leaks and benign esophageal perforations. Ann Surg 2014;259(5):852–60.
9. Kamarajah SK, Bundred J, Spence G, et al. Critical appraisal of the impact of oesophageal stents in the management of oesophageal anastomotic leaks and benign oesophageal perforations: an updated systematic review. World J Surg 2020;44(4):1173–89.
10. Odell JA, DeVault KR. Extended stent usage for persistent esophageal leak: should there be limits? Ann Thorac Surg 2010;90(5):1707–8.
11. Freeman RK, Ascioti AJ, Dake M, et al. An assessment of the optimal time for removal of esophageal stents used in the treatment of an esophageal anastomotic leak or perforation. Ann Thorac Surg 2015;100(2):422–8.
12. Whitelocke D, Maddaus M, Andrade R, et al. Gastro-aortic fistula: a rare and lethal complication of esophageal stenting after esophagectomy. J Thorac Cardiovasc Surg 2010;140(3):e49–50.

13. Jena A, Chandnani S, Jain S, et al. Efficacy of endoscopic over-the-scope clip fixation for preventing migration of self-expandable metal stents: a systematic review and meta-analysis. Surgical Endoscopy and Other Interventional Techniques 2023;37(5): 3410–8.

14. Kantsevoy SV, Bitner M. Esophageal stent fixation with endoscopic suturing device (with video). Gastrointest Endosc 2012;76(6):1251–5.

15. Sharaiha RZ, Kumta NA, DeFilippis EM, et al. A large multicenter experience with endoscopic suturing for management of gastrointestinal defects and stent anchorage in 122 patients: a retrospective review. J Clin Gastroenterol 2016;50(5):388–92.

16. Gangwani MK, Ahmed Z, Aziz M, et al. Comparing endoscopic suture vs clip vs no intervention in esophageal stent migration: a network meta-analysis. Tech Innovat Gastroi 2024;26(2):145–52.

17. Ong GKB, Freeman RK, Ascioti AJ, et al. Patient outcomes after stent failure for the treatment of acute esophageal perforation. Ann Thorac Surg 2018; 106(3):830–5.

18. Binmoeller KF, Grimm H, Soehendra N. Endoscopic closure of a perforation using metallic clips after snare excision of a gastric leiomyoma. Gastrointest Endosc 1993;39(2):172–4.

19. Qadeer MA, Dumot JA, Vargo JJ, et al. Endoscopic clips for closing esophageal perforations: case report and pooled analysis. Gastrointest Endosc 2007;66(3):605–11.

20. Manta R, Manno M, Bertani H, et al. Endoscopic treatment of gastrointestinal fistulas using an over-the-scope clip (OTSC) device: case series from a tertiary referral center. Endoscopy 2011;43(6):545–8.

21. Haito-Chavez Y, Law JK, Kratt T, et al. International multicenter experience with an over-the-scope clipping device for endoscopic management of GI defects (with video). Gastrointest Endosc 2014;80(4):610–22.

22. Mennigen R, Senninger N, Laukoetter MG. Novel treatment options for perforations of the upper gastrointestinal tract: endoscopic vacuum therapy and over-the-scope clips. World J Gastroenterol 2014;20(24):7767–76.

23. Voermans RP, Le Moine O, von Renteln D, et al. Efficacy of endoscopic closure of acute perforations of the gastrointestinal tract. Clin Gastroenterol Hepatol 2012;10(6):603–8.

24. Lazar G, Paszt A, Man E. Role of endoscopic clipping in the treatment of oesophageal perforations. World J Gastrointest Endosc 2016;8(1):13–22.

25. Venturi ML, Attinger CE, Mesbahi AN, et al. Mechanisms and clinical applications of the vacuum-assisted closure (VAC) Device: a review. Am J Clin Dermatol 2005;6(3):185–94.

26. Moore CB, Almoghrabi O, Hofstetter W, et al. Endoluminal wound vac: an evolving role in treatment of esophageal perforation. J Vis Surg 2020;6.

27. Brangewitz M, Voigtlander T, Helfritz FA, et al. Endoscopic closure of esophageal intrathoracic leaks: stent versus endoscopic vacuum-assisted closure, a retrospective analysis. Endoscopy 2013;45(6):433–8.

28. Loske G, Schorsch T, Muller C. Intraluminal and intracavitary vacuum therapy for esophageal leakage: a new endoscopic minimally invasive approach. Endoscopy 2011;43(6):540–4.

29. Ahrens M, Schulte T, Egberts J, et al. Drainage of esophageal leakage using endoscopic vacuum therapy: a prospective pilot study. Endoscopy 2010;42(9):693–8.

30. Schorsch T, Muller C, Loske G. [Endoscopic vacuum therapy of perforations and anastomotic insufficiency of the esophagus]. Chirurg 2014;85(12):1081–93. Endoskopische Vakuumtherapie von Perforationen und Anastomoseninsuffizienzen des Osophagus.

31. Still S, Mencio M, Ontiveros E, et al. Primary and rescue endoluminal vacuum therapy in the management of esophageal perforations and leaks. Ann Thorac Cardiovasc Surg 2018;24(4):173–9.

32. Jung CFM, Müller-Dornieden A, Gaedcke J, et al. Impact of endoscopic vacuum therapy with low negative pressure for esophageal perforations and postoperative anastomotic esophageal leaks. Digestion 2021;102(3):469–79.

33. Bludau M, Fuchs HF, Herbold T, et al. Results of endoscopic vacuum-assisted closure device for treatment of upper GI leaks. Surg Endosc 2018; 32(4):1906–14.

34. Kuehn F, Schiffmann L, Janisch F, et al. Surgical endoscopic vacuum therapy for defects of the upper gastrointestinal tract. J Gastrointest Surg 2016; 20(2):237–43.

35. Newton NJ, Sharrock A, Rickard R, et al. Systematic review of the use of endo-luminal topical negative pressure in oesophageal leaks and perforations. Dis Esophagus 2017;30(3).

36. Leeds SG, Mencio M, Ontiveros E, et al. Endoluminal vacuum therapy: how i do it. J Gastrointest Surg 2019;23(5):1037–43.

37. Mencio MA, Ontiveros E, Burdick JS, et al. Use of a novel technique to manage gastrointestinal leaks with endoluminal negative pressure: a single institution experience. Surg Endosc 2018;32(7):3349–56.

38. Bludau M, Holscher AH, Herbold T, et al. Management of upper intestinal leaks using an endoscopic vacuum-assisted closure system (E-VAC). Surg Endosc 2014;28(3):896–901.

39. Henderson JB, Sorser SA, Atia AN, et al. Repair of esophageal perforations using a novel endoscopic suturing system. Gastrointest Endosc 2014;80(3): 535–7.

40. Kurian AA, Bhayani NH, Reavis K, et al. Endoscopic suture repair of full-thickness esophagotomy during per-oral esophageal myotomy for achalasia. Surg Endosc 2013;27(10):3910.

41. Raju GS, Thompson C, Zwischenberger JB. Emerging endoscopic options in the management of esophageal leaks (videos). Gastrointest Endosc 2005;62(2):278–86.

42. Al Ghossaini N, Lucidarme D, Bulois P. Endoscopic treatment of iatrogenic gastrointestinal perforations: an overview. Dig Liver Dis 2014;46(3):195–203.

43. Freeman RK, Herrera A, Ascioti AJ, et al. A propensity-matched comparison of cost and outcomes after esophageal stent placement or primary surgical repair for iatrogenic esophageal perforation. J Thorac Cardiovasc Surg 2015;149(6):1550–5.

44. Ben-David K, Behrns K, Hochwald S, et al. Esophageal perforation management using a multidisciplinary minimally invasive treatment algorithm. J Am Coll Surg 2014;218(4):768–74.

45. D'Cunha J, Rueth NM, Groth SS, et al. Esophageal stents for anastomotic leaks and perforations. J Thorac Cardiovasc Surg 2011;142(1):39–46 e1.

46. Freeman RK, Ascioti AJ, Giannini T, et al. Analysis of unsuccessful esophageal stent placements for esophageal perforation, fistula, or anastomotic leak. Ann Thorac Surg 2012;94(3):959–64. discussion 964-5.

Management of Complications After Per Oral Endoscopic Myotomy

Francois Khazoom, MD, MSc[a], Brian E. Louie, MD, MPH, MHA, FRCSC[a],*

KEYWORDS

- Per oral endoscopic myotomy (POEM) • Complications • Achalasia • Motility disorders

KEY POINTS

- Understanding mechanisms of per oral endoscopic myotomy (POEM) complication is key to their prevention.
- Intraoperative complications are best prevented and can be managed with simple endoscopic procedures.
- Short-term postoperative complications are infrequent.
- Long-term postoperative complications and their consequences remain to be defined.

INTRODUCTION

Achalasia is the most common esophageal motor disorder in North America, characterized by absent or ineffective peristalsis and failure of the lower esophageal sphincter (LES) to relax in response to deglutition. As its pathogenesis involves the destruction of the neural plexus in the esophageal wall, normal peristalsis cannot be restored. Therefore, the goals of surgical treatment are two-fold: first, perform a myotomy of the LES to allow esophageal emptying by gravity; and second, minimize gastroesophageal reflux through a fundoplication or proton-pump inhibitors (PPIs).

Per oral endoscopic myotomy (POEM) was first performed in humans in 2008.[1] Since then, the procedure has been widely adopted in North America, being performed in multiple centers as an alternative to balloon dilatation and laparoscopic Heller myotomy. With literature emerging comparing POEM with Heller myotomy or pneumatic dilation,[2,3] the American College of Gastroenterology recommends POEM as the treatment of choice of type III achalasia and as an equivalent alternative to laparoscopic Heller myotomy for types I and II.

As the role of POEM in the treatment of achalasia becomes more and more defined, the number of procedures performed is expected to increase in the future. With this in mind, understanding complications, their prevention, and their management becomes paramount. This article describes complications of POEM, including perioperative, early, and late adverse events, with an emphasis on prevention and management.

INTRAOPERATIVE ADVERSE EVENTS
Mucosal Injury

Along the length of the myotomy, the mucosa is the only barrier between the esophageal lumen and the mediastinum. The rate of mucosal injury in POEM ranges from 1.6% to 26%.[4] Unrecognized mucosal injury at the level of the myotomy essentially represents free esophageal perforation and can have disastrous consequences, such as mediastinitis, empyema, and death.[5] The key to minimizing morbidity is early recognition during the procedure, reinforcing the need to perform a

[a] Division of Thoracic Surgery, Swedish Cancer Institute and Medical Center, 1101 Madison Street, Suite 900, Seattle, WA 90814, USA
* Corresponding author.
E-mail address: brian.louie@swedish.org

Thorac Surg Clin 34 (2024) 341–353
https://doi.org/10.1016/j.thorsurg.2024.05.006
1547-4127/24/© 2024 Elsevier Inc. All rights reserved, including those for text and data mining, AI training, and similar technologies.

second-look endoscopy where second-look endoscopy allows recognition of an addition 11% of mucosal injuries.[6] Although the most common mechanism is cautery injury, mechanical injury because of excessive torquing of the scope in the tunnel or across the mucosotomy site may also occur. Endoscopic signs include visualization of a mucosal hematoma, visualization of a cautery burn in the form of blanching mucosa, visualization of a full-thickness mucosal injury, or loss of ability to inflate the tunnel with CO_2 during the procedure.[7]

Mucosal injuries most commonly occur at the gastroesophageal junction (GEJ) but can occur anywhere along the tunnel. At the GEJ, the mucosa and the muscle layers are in close proximity, making dissection of the submucosal plane more challenging. In addition, the increased tone of the LES in achalasia creates an angle that narrows the lumen, thereby decreasing the distance between the muscle layer and the mucosa. Submucosal fibrosis is commonly encountered at this level but also occurs because of prior interventions, such as pneumatic dilation or botulinum toxin injection. Prior surgical interventions, such as Heller myotomy or POEM, can also create risk. Other risk factors are related to difficult anatomy, including (1) sigmoid esophagus; (2) tunnel length greater than 13 cm; and (3) prior stent placement.[4]

Key principles to prevent mucosal injuries are as follows: (1) liberal use of saline injection in the submucosal plane to lift mucosa away from the site of dissection; (2) operating in SM3 territory right on the circular muscle (**Fig. 1**); (3) sharp dissection with short bursts using cut as opposed to coagulation settings to minimize energy dispersion; (4)

widening the tunnel to improve working space (**Fig. 2**); (5) careful anticipatory hemostasis to preserve good visualization of the submucosal plane; and (6) when working at the GEJ or where significant submucosal fibrosis, initiation of the myotomy before completion of the tunnel may improve working space.[7,8]

Partial-thickness mucosal injuries away from the myotomy site are generally best managed expectantly. When these injuries occur within the myotomy region, they are best closed primarily with endoscopic clips to reapproximate healthy mucosa together, as delayed thermal injury progression to full-thickness injury has been described.[7] Straightforward full-thickness mucosal injuries should be closed primarily with endoscopic clips, irrespective of their location with respect to the myotomy. Large mucosal injuries or those associated with significant submucosal fibrosis may prevent reapproximation with endoscopic clips. In these situations, closure with an endoscopic suturing device may be required.[9,10] Only rarely will endoscopic closure not be feasible; in these cases, fibrin glue has been described as safe and effective.[11,12] Use of a covered stent should be avoided unless absolutely necessary owing to the high risk of migration when placed in a dilated esophagus.

Bleeding

Bleeding during POEM can be encountered during any step of the procedure. It most commonly occurs during submucosal tunneling near the GEJ, where submucosal vessels are generally denser and where limited working space favors inadvertent avulsion of these vessels. Most bleeding events are minor and represent a threat to adequate visualization and exposure, predisposing to more vessel

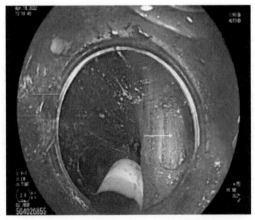

Fig. 1. Operating in SM3 territory (as close as possible to the circular muscle, *yellow arrow*) allows dissection as far as possible from the mucosa (*red arrow*) and avoids energy transfer.

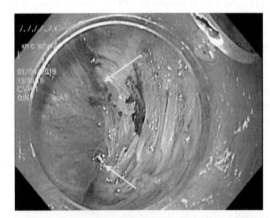

Fig. 2. Widening the tunnel at the gastroesophageal junction (*yellow arrow*) allows improved working space to minimize energy transfer to the mucosa.

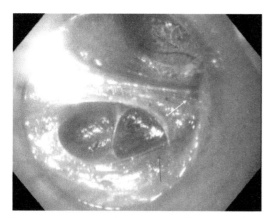

Fig. 3. Bridging vessels (*red* and *yellow arrows*) between the mucosa and the muscular layer. Isolation of a vessel to facilitate coagulation.

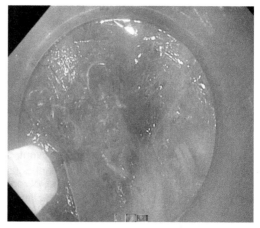

Fig. 4. Liberal use of submucosal injection allows one to lift the mucosa away from the site of dissection when isolating a vessel for coagulation.

avulsion and mucosal injuries, rather than a hemodynamically significant problem. In a large series of 1826 patients, only 2 patients had significant bleeding that required abortion of the procedure and invasive hemostatic methods.[13] Patients on anticoagulation and those with advanced achalasia are at increased risk owing to hypertrophied submucosal vessels and tortuosity of the esophagus.[14]

Prevention starts with adequate cessation of anticoagulation preprocedure. As well, the site of mucosotomy should be carefully inspected, and a relatively avascular site should be chosen with adequate saline injection to widen the submucosal plane. During submucosal tunneling, sources of bleeding include submucosal vessels bridging the muscle layer and the mucosa, vessels located on either edge of the tunnel, and large submucosal vessels located near the GEJ (**Fig. 3**).[7,15] Preemptive coagulation of bridging vessels is key to preventing troublesome bleeding. This can be accomplished by using coagulation settings on the knife or a coagulating grasper for larger vessels. Ideally, submucosal injection and dissection of the vessel away from the mucosa prevent thermal spread (**Fig. 4**). In addition, the tunnel should be widened to a size that allows the advancement of the endoscope without resistance to avoid the avulsion of vessels on either side of the tunnel.

When significant bleeding is encountered, application of pressure using the cap of the endoscope and gentle suctioning often allows enough tamponade to localize the bleeding and coagulate it (**Fig. 5**). If localization fails, the likely bleeding site can be injected with saline to attempt further tamponade. As well, the tunnel can be filled with water using the jet function of the endoscope, and the bleeding site can be further localized under water. Widening the tunnel is also a key maneuver

that allows improved working space, thereby decreasing the risk of mucosal injury and improving visualization. Once the bleeding site is localized and dissected away from the mucosa, it can be safely coagulated. If the bleeding site cannot be safely dissected off the mucosa, it can be grasped precisely and lifted away from the mucosa with a coagulation grasper.

Insufflation-Related Events

Insufflation-related events are common occurrences after POEM, and only those requiring an additional intervention should be characterized as true adverse events. Pannu and colleagues[16] prospectively studied computed tomographic (CT) esophagogram findings after POEM and found

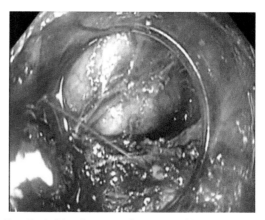

Fig. 5. A bleeding vessel compromising view and obscuring dissection planes. The cap was subsequently used to put pressure on the vessel while dissecting the vessel away from the mucosa for coagulation. (Image courtesy of Dr. Christy Dunst.)

high rates of pneumomediastinum (86%), pneumoperitoneum (66%), subcutaneous emphysema (52.4%), retroperitoneal air (38%), and pneumothorax (19%). Pneumopericardium was a rare event at 2.4%. However, none of these insufflation-related findings required a reintervention. A large retrospective study showed that the incidence of true adverse events related to insufflation was 1.6% with capnoperitoneum (1.2%), capnothorax (0.32%) and capnomediastinum (0.1%) being the most frequent when the definition of an event is based on the need additional intervention.[13]

Prevention strategies include the use of CO_2 instead of room air, avoidance of a full-thickness myotomy, and avoidance of excessive insufflation when a full-thickness myotomy has been recognized. Pneumothorax can be avoided by respecting the above principles and promptly recognizing inadvertent entry in the mediastinum. The abdomen should be palpated serially during the procedure to detect tense pneumoperitoneum, which would lead to postoperative discomfort. Pneumopericardium can be theoretically avoided by avoiding a frankly anterior myotomy, respecting the 2 o'clock or 5 o'clock principles.[17]

Management is most often expectant as CO_2 is highly blood soluble and rapidly reabsorbed. Clinically significant pneumoperitoneum can be decompressed with a Veress needle, which is left in place until the procedure is completed. Pneumothorax rarely requires pleural drainage unless clinical instability occurs; in this case, drainage is required to continue the procedure. Pneumopericardium has been described as a rare cause of intraoperative cardiac arrest.[18,19] Both reported events were related to technical factors, including the use of air insufflation instead of CO_2[18] and unusual fibrosis of muscle layers with pericardium.[19] In both cases the procedure was aborted, and cardiac arrest was managed as per Advanced Cardiovascular Life Support guidelines. Pneumopericardium was recognized postoperatively. In the rare event where clinical instability is thought to be related to insufflation complications, such as tension capnothorax or tension capnopericardium, a brief interruption of the procedure without insufflation whatsoever generally suffices to reestablish clinical stability and continue the procedure. When instability progresses to cardiac arrest, bilateral chest tubes and subxiphoid pericardial window can be lifesaving.

EARLY POSTOPERATIVE COMPLICATIONS
Delayed Intratunnel Bleeding

Although intraoperative bleeding is a frequent event with little consequences if managed appropriately, postoperative intratunnel bleeding has been reported in 0.3% to 5% of patients undergoing POEM.[7,20,21] Delayed intratunnel bleeding can have clinically significant consequences, such as upper gastrointestinal (GI) bleeding, dysphagia, chest pain, hemorrhagic shock, and infection of the submucosal hematoma. Prevention of such adverse events starts with adequate cessation of anticoagulation and careful hemostasis during the procedure. However, early diagnosis and management may be challenging because blood generally accumulates slowly until intratunnel pressure increases and causes pain. An intramural hematoma usually forms and causes bleeding to stop, but ongoing bleeding may rupture the mucosotomy closure or partial-thickness mucosal injury and lead to upper GI bleeding. With initiation of oral intake, and perhaps with concomitant unrecognized mucosal injuries, the hematoma may become infected.

Wang and colleagues[20] reported a case series of 22 patients with delayed bleeding after an endoscopic submucosal tunneling procedure, 17 of which had intratunnel bleeding. The most common presenting symptoms were hematemesis (72.7%), fever (36.4%), and melena (18.2%). One-third of patients had concomitant mucosal injury, which led to a persistent fistula in 20% of patients overall. The tunnel infection rate was 9.1%. Most patients had a hemoglobin drop of more than 20 g/L at presentation. More than half of the patients were diagnosed after discharge (mean, 5.3 days) and required readmission. Rarely, intratunnel bleeding may progress through the myotomy into the mediastinum and rupture the pleura, leading to hemothorax.[22] This complication is best diagnosed with CT scan, which will show an intramural collection with heterogeneous enhancement between 35 and 70 Hounsfield units. Confirmation is then obtained with an esophagogastroduodenoscopy (EGD).

Initial management of intratunnel hematoma includes pain control, resuscitation, intravenous antibiotics, and nutritional support. Small, completely asymptomatic submucosal hematoma without evidence of active bleeding is generally managed expectantly. Endoscopic evacuation of the hematoma and hemostasis is mandatory for large, symptomatic hematoma and/or evidence of active submucosal tunnel bleeding. This is often a laborious procedure because of a limited working space filled with clots (**Fig. 6**). The mucosotomy site is reopened; the tunnel is entered, and clots are evacuated. Common bleeding sites, such as myotomy edges and submucosal vessels, are carefully inspected along the entire length of the tunnel. These are coagulated respecting principles outlined in the acute bleeding section. Copious

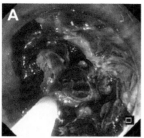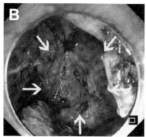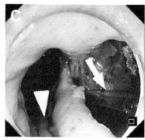

Fig. 6. Delayed intratunnel bleeding with large clots in the tunnel (*A*). View of the tunnel after clot removal, which transformed into a cavity (*B, yellow arrows*). Placement of intracavitary nasogastric tube (*arrow*) and feeding tube (*arrow- head*) (*C*). (Reprinted with permission from Wang L, Liu ZQ, Zhang JY, et al. Management of delayed bleeding of upper gastrointestinal endoscopic submucosal tunneling procedures: a retrospective single-center analysis and brief meta-analysis. *Journal of Gastroenterology and Hepatology (Australia)*. 2023;38(12):2174-2184. https://doi.org/10.1111/jgh.16361.)

water irrigation in the tunnel is also helpful in visualizing bleeding sites. Further tamponade of the tunnel with a Blakemore tube has been described, but this practice carries a high risk of mucosal perforation with a myotomy in place and is discouraged. Repeat closure of the original mucosotomy can be challenging in delayed presentations and may require adjuncts for difficult closures, such as over-the-scope clips or endoscopic suturing devices.

Infection of the hematoma requires prompt source control in the form of endoscopic drainage, debridement, and copious irrigation. Once this is achieved, an important decision is whether the mucosotomy should be closed. Closure of the mucosotomy is advised in the patient who presents in a nondelayed fashion with acceptable tissue quality. For the delayed presentation with friable tissues and extensive infection of the tunnel, leaving a nasogastric tube drainage in the tunnel cavity has been described. Placement of a nasojejunal feeding tube is always wise in this context to optimize nutrition in a mucosotomy closure that is at higher risk of failure (see **Fig. 6**).[7,20]

Failure of the Mucosotomy Closure

Mucosotomy closure is one of the most critical parts of the procedure. Failure of the mucosotomy closure recognized postoperatively is rare, estimated at less than 1% in most studies.[15,21] Prevention of this adverse event starts with preemptive intravenous steroids after induction of anesthesia to decrease mucosal edema and thereby facilitate closure. In addition, the mucosotomy should be performed strategically respecting the following principles: first, the mucosotomy should be performed 5 cm proximal to the start of the myotomy to avoid full-thickness perforation in the event of mucosotomy failure; second,

the mucosotomy should be performed in a way that facilitates endoscopic closure. It is the authors' preference to perform the mucosotomy parallel to the long axis of the esophagus and plan its length to be just long enough to accommodate the therapeutic scope.[8]

Another important principle is to ensure a complete myotomy to relieve any distal obstruction that would impair healing of the mucosotomy. After the procedure, the mucosotomy is closed by applying the first endoclip a few millimeters distal to the mucosotomy to create a mucosal ridge. Successive clips are then applied from distal to proximal, apposing mucosa on each edge.[8] An endoscopic suturing device is an alternative option for mucosotomy closure. A retrospective study showed no difference in postoperative mucosotomy failure between endoscopic suturing and endoclip application, with the former having higher cost and closure time.[10] Endoscopic suturing closure may be best reserved for patients with difficult closures related to mucosal edema or when the mucosotomy orientation does not allow clip closure. When the mucosotomy is inadvertently too wide for reapproximation, clipping the mucosa on the muscular wall of the esophagus may be the best strategy to promote healing. Fibrin glue has also been described. Stents as a means of primary mucosotomy closure are best avoided, as they carry concerns of migration and radial ischemia.

Failure of the mucosotomy closure that is recognized postoperatively can present with a contained leak, a leak into the tunnel leading to intramural esophageal contamination/abscess, full-thickness perforation with mediastinitis, or free perforation in either pleural space. Although patients with an asymptomatic contained leak may be treated successfully with a trial of NPO (nothing by mouth) and antibiotics, an endoscopy

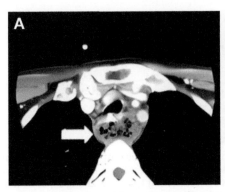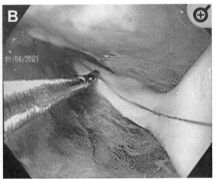

Fig. 7. Intratunnel Jackson-Pratt. The patient underwent Z-POEM and presented with a retroesophageal collection (*A, arrow*). An intracavitary Jackson-Pratt was placed (*B*). (Reprinted with permission from Daza Castro EM, Fuentes CF, Córdoba Guzmán AC, et al. Multimodal Endoscopic Management of Esophageal Perforations as a Complication of Peroral Endoscopic Myotomy for a Zenker's Diverticulum. *ACG Case Rep J.* 2023;10(6):e01059. https://doi.org/10.14309/crj.0000000000001059.)

should be performed to evaluate the site of the leak and the ability to further close it endoscopically. When these are discovered early enough (usually within 24 hours), little inflammation is expected on the mucosotomy site, and endoscopic closure with clips or endosuturing can be achieved.[23] After 2 to 3 days, inflammation of the mucosa and contamination of the tunnel, mediastinum, and pleural spaces may occur.

When contamination is limited to the tunnel, appropriate source control can be achieved by endoscopic washout and irrigation of the tunnel. In a recent paper on Z-POEM, placing a nasal Jackson-Pratt in the defect was used and could be adapted to drain the POEM tunnel (**Fig. 7**).[24] Adequate nutrition should be maintained with a nasogastric feeding tube or a feeding jejunostomy. The Jackson-Pratt can then be withdrawn serially until the tunnel has sealed. At this point, if a persistent mucosal defect is present, it can be managed with an endoluminal wound vac until healthy granulation tissue reepithelialization occurs.[24]

Any associated pleural effusion, even if considered reactive, should be drained to prevent bacterial translocation and empyema. If there is free perforation with significant mediastinal and/or pleural contamination, the patient should undergo thoracotomy, decortication, mediastinal debridement, and primary repair with muscle flap reinforcement, if feasible. If not feasible, options include a covered stent combined with video-assisted thoracic surgery (VATS) decortication/mediastinal debridement or esophagectomy with or without reconstruction. Factors influencing which approach to choose include patient's comorbidities, the severity of esophageal dilatation and tortuosity, and whether end-stage achalasia is present.

SHORT-TERM COMPLICATIONS
Recurrent Dysphagia: Reflux Stricture, Incomplete Myotomy, Food Impaction

The differential diagnosis of early recurrent dysphagia after POEM includes incomplete myotomy, reflux stricture, excessive scarring at the myotomy site, food impaction, or incorrect initial diagnosis. Recurrent dysphagia that occurs later in the disease course should raise concerns for progression to end-stage achalasia and esophageal malignancy, whether adenocarcinoma from longstanding clinically silent reflux or squamous cell carcinoma in association with achalasia.

In general, recurrent dysphagia after surgical treatment of achalasia should prompt a repeat upper endoscopy, an upper GI contrast study, a high-resolution manometry, and possibly a pH study.[25] Consideration may also be given to EndoFlip assessment. Any stricture should be biopsied to rule out malignancy.

Prevention of early recurrent dysphagia requires a fine balance between the risk of reflux-associated stricture and incomplete myotomy. Although attempting the most minimal myotomy may help prevent reflux and a subsequent stricture, this strategy would also potentially increase the risk of incomplete myotomy. Use of the functional luminal imaging probe (EndoFlip) may allow more precise measurement of distensibility at the level of the LES before and after the myotomy, and potentially allowing one to perform a more limited myotomy without compromising postoperative improvement of dysphagia.[8,26,27] This ultimately may mitigate the risk of reflux as well, allowing for shorter myotomies. Although promising, these assumptions remain theoretic, and further data are required to support a strong recommendation for routine EndoFlip use during POEM. Reflux-related stricture may also be prevented with routine use of PPIs until a postoperative pH study off PPI confirms the absence of acid reflux.[28]

Treatment is dictated by the cause of postoperative dysphagia. The incidence of peptic stricture after POEM is not well characterized but is generally considered a rare event. Peptic strictures should be initially treated with a combination of dilatation and PPI therapy. Peptic stricture recurring after dilatation while on PPI therapy should be considered for a partial fundoplication with the objective of improving reflux control and promoting healing. Esophagectomy is the treatment of choice for a nondilatable stricture downstream of an atonic esophagus.

Early recurrent dysphagia without evidence of a peptic stricture should raise concerns regarding excessive fibrosis at the myotomy site or incomplete myotomy. Repeat manometry and EndoFlip may help document these entities objectively, but it is only at reoperation that they can be differentiated definitively. Initial treatment options that have been documented as safe include small-caliber dilation (20 mm or less), pneumatic dilatation, repeat POEM, or Heller myotomy. Although pneumatic dilatation is a well-established treatment option after a failed Heller myotomy,[29] few studies have documented its use after POEM. Van Hoeij and colleagues[30] have attempted pneumatic dilatation in 15 patients who had failed POEM and reported a low success rate of 20%. In another study by Werner and colleagues,[31] none of the 4 patients who underwent pneumatic dilation after POEM had a meaningful response.

Repeat POEM for recurrent dysphagia has been characterized by Tyberg and colleagues[32] as part of an international registry of redo POEM. Among 46 patients, technical success was achieved in all, and clinical success was achieved in 85% of patients as defined by an Eckardt score of 3 or less. Adverse events were all related to intraoperative bleeding at 18%, and all episodes were controlled endoscopically during the procedure.[32] A critical technical component of redo POEM is to perform the tunnel and myotomy in the opposite orientation (anterior vs posterior) of what was performed during the initial procedure, thus avoiding a scarred submucosal plane.[8,32] Interestingly, the data on repeat POEM appear to be associated with fewer adverse events than repeat Heller myotomy. Possible explanations are the ability to create a tunnel and myotomy in a virgin plane in the opposite orientation and avoidance of intra-abdominal adhesions.[32,33] The ability to use a virgin plane in a redo procedure is also a compelling reason POEM is generally favored over redo Heller myotomy if the patient is thought to have an incomplete myotomy or excessive scarring without issues with the fundoplication.[32]

The option of laparoscopic Heller myotomy as a rescue procedure after failed POEM has not been studied well. A few case reports have documented its safety in a small number of patients.[34] This option may be more compelling for the rare patient with recurrent dysphagia associated with reflux refractory to PPIs. It should not be the first option overall, especially if the initial POEM was performed anteriorly.

LONGER-TERM COMPLICATIONS
Gastroesophageal Reflux Disease/Esophagitis

One of the main criticisms of POEM has been its high incidence of postoperative gastroesophageal reflux disease (GERD), which has been attributed to the lack of an antireflux procedure after the myotomy. Although postoperative reflux has been consistently higher in POEM compared with laparoscopic Heller myotomy,[2] POEM does have some theoretic advantages compared with Heller myotomy that might minimize postoperative reflux. These include the following: (1) lack of dissection of the GEJ and preservation of the angle of His; (2) ability to divide circular muscle only; and (3) preservation of the sling fibers of the cardia. This suggests that the ability to perform an antireflux procedure during a Heller myotomy is an important factor to prevent GERD. On the other hand, it also suggests that if a myotomy only is to be performed and fundoplication omitted, POEM does have some theoretic advantages.

The reported incidence of GERD after POEM is heavily dependent on the use of objective studies, such as pH testing or endoscopy, in the assessment of reflux. Indeed, a correlation between GERD symptoms and pH testing does not seem to exist after POEM,[35] suggesting that many asymptomatic patients will have objective evidence of GERD if testing is undertaken. Bearing this in mind, it is not surprising that studies using routine pH testing and endoscopy at follow-up have reported higher rates of GERD, which were between 40% and 57.8%.[7,36,37] More precisely, in a recent study, rates of subjective, objective, and severe GERD, defined as a DeMeester score of greater than 50 or grade D esophagitis, were 38.8%, 50.5%, and 19.2%, respectively.[38] This study has also shown that 24% of asymptomatic patients had objective evidence of GERD after POEM. Until long-term sequelae of long-standing clinically silent reflux are further defined, this argues for routine postoperative pH testing and follow-up endoscopy after POEM.

Well-established patient-related risk factors for GERD after POEM include obesity, female gender, normal esophageal diameter, and LES pressure less than 45 mm Hg on preoperative manometry.[38] Procedure factors that may impact post-POEM reflux are as follows: (1) myotomy length; (2) location of the myotomy (posterior vs anterior); and (3) thickness of the myotomy (circular only vs full). A recent randomized study of 94 patients with type II achalasia has shown that a short myotomy (3–4 cm on the esophageal side and 2–3 cm on the gastric side) had decreased esophageal acid exposure.[39] The location of the myotomy has theoretic differences in the risk of reflux, where an anterior myotomy may lead to less reflux owing to preservation of the posterior oblique fibers, which maintain the angle of His. Although Ramchandani and colleagues[40] showed that a posterior myotomy led to more abnormal DeMeester scores compared with an anterior myotomy, both groups had a long myotomy (12–13 cm), and length was not well balanced between groups. A recent well-powered randomized controlled trial showed that myotomy location had no impact on post-POEM GERD.[41] In both groups, the post-POEM DeMeester score was greater than 14.72 in 42% to 49% of patients, and PPI use at 1 year was 20%. Results were similar at 2 years, although more patients had to be placed on PPI in the anterior group (41% vs 15%, nonsignificant).[17] This corroborates the high-acid-reflux rate after POEM and the fact that most patients will either be asymptomatic or respond to PPI therapy. The thickness of the myotomy is also a subject of debate, where a full-thickness myotomy has been associated with higher rates of reflux,[42] whereas other studies have shown no association.[43] A recent retrospective study has shown that preservation of the sling fibers (**Fig. 8**) by performing the gastric aspect of the myotomy on the lesser curve decreased Los Angeles (LA) grade C or D esophagitis (18.1% vs 44.1%).[44]

It is important to consider that, although little high-quality data exist to guide the technical aspects of POEM, the priority in achalasia surgery remains palliation of dysphagia, with prevention of reflux being a secondary goal. Based on the above data, it appears that performing a shorter myotomy (3–4 cm on the esophagus and 2–3 cm on the stomach), performing a partial-thickness circular myotomy, performing the myotomy anteriorly, and preserving the sling fibers are reasonable attempts to minimize post-POEM reflux without compromising on dysphagia palliation, whether based on data or theoretic concepts.

Most patients with reflux after POEM will respond to PPI therapy. In patients with PPI-refractory symptoms, delayed gastric emptying should be ruled out, and consideration should be given to partial fundoplication after POEM.

Esophageal Pseudodiverticulum

One of the proposed mechanisms for POEM failure is the development of pseudodiverticulum at the site of myotomy. This has been defined as a wide diverticulum (>2 cm) myotomy or luminal dilatation greater than 50% of the remaining esophagus at the site of the myotomy.[45] Interestingly, this complication appears to be more frequent after Heller myotomy with fundoplication compared with POEM, patients with type III achalasia, and patients with greater initial myotomy.[45] These risk factors are all related to increased intraluminal pressure leading to outpouching of the mucosa at the myotomy site, whether related to the relative obstruction created by fundoplication or spasms of type III achalasia. Myotomy length was not associated with pseudodiverticulum, but an experimental model showed longer length to contribute to pseudodiverticulum formation, in accordance with Laplace's law.[46]

The development of a pseudodiverticulum has been associated with higher rates of clinical failure after myotomy (up to 56%), occurring at a median time of 51 months after myotomy.[45] Patients generally have higher dysphagia and regurgitation scores, which translate into a poorer quality of life.[45] Because of the lack of standardized follow-up after myotomy for achalasia, the true denominator of patients developing a pseudodiverticulum after myotomy is unknown. This entity is best left alone in asymptomatic patients. There is no literature guiding treatments of symptomatic patients. Mildly symptomatic patients should be treated with lifestyle modifications. Patients with significant recurrent dysphagia and regurgitation should be treated with surgery. Options include laparoscopic diverticulectomy and ensuring a complete myotomy distal, or esophagectomy.

Progressive Esophageal Dilatation

One of the proposed advantages of POEM is its ability to perform a long myotomy minimally invasively, which has been adopted by some for spastic esophageal disorders.[47] However, pushing the above principles to the extreme, one could hypothesize that performing an overly long myotomy for disorders with high esophageal body pressures would favor progressive esophageal dilatation, complete dysfunction, and, at the extreme of the spectrum, a totally ischemic esophagus from

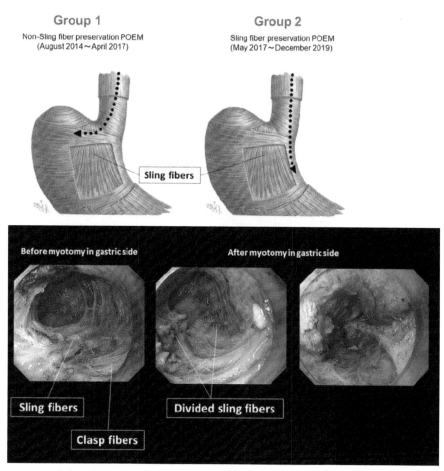

Fig. 8. Preservation of sling fibers is thought to reduce post-POEM GERD. (Reprinted with permission from Shiwaku H, Inoue H, Shiwaku A, Okada H, Hasegawa S. Safety and effectiveness of sling fiber preservation POEM to reduce severe post-procedural erosive esophagitis. *Surg Endosc.* 2022;36(6):4255-4264. https://doi.org/10.1007/s00464-021-08763-w.)

venous congestion. Although this has not been reported yet in the literature after POEM, the senior author has experienced such a situation where the patient ultimately needed an esophagectomy. The patient was a 62-year-old woman with progressive dysphagia diagnosed with type II achalasia based on manometry and timed barium swallow. The patient had undergone a 21-cm myotomy (2-cm gastric, 19-cm esophageal) at an outside institution. Postoperatively, although no reflux symptoms were present, she developed a reflux stricture at the GEJ, which was ultimately dilated to 20 mm. The patient was placed on PPI twice daily but had deteriorating GERD symptoms and progressive esophageal dilatation despite maximal PPI therapy. With worsening reflux, progressive esophageal dilatation, and dysphagia, the patient ultimately required esophagectomy (**Fig. 9**). This case exemplifies that although

esophagectomy for benign disease is often considered last resort, the development of a peptic stricture in the face of a massively dilated, myotomized esophagus often leads to a vicious circle where dilating the stricture will worsen GERD and the low clearance ability of the myotomized esophagus will not be able to compensate, ultimately making esophagectomy a necessity.

A parallel can be made when reviewing the early literature of long transthoracic myotomies done for spastic esophageal disorders. Nastos and colleagues[48] have published their results of 16 patients undergoing long myotomy for esophageal spastic disorders. Symptom improvement was minimal, and 4 ultimately needed surgery for progressive esophageal dilatation and dysfunction. Three of these patients had esophagectomy without symptomatic improvement afterward.

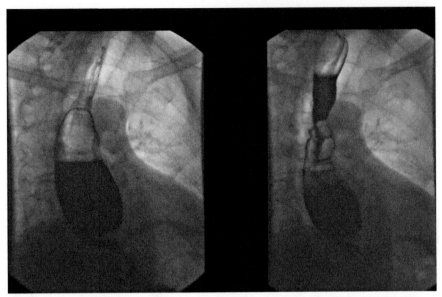

Fig. 9. Progressive esophageal dilatation after a 21-cm myotomy for type II achalasia. The patient ultimately required esophagectomy owing to progressive dilatation and PPI-refractory GERD.

The investigators concluded that esophageal spastic disorders, especially without a diverticulum, respond poorly to surgery and require more invasive revisional procedures. No data have been published so far, and long-term follow-up will either confirm or refute whether a parallel exists with POEM.

Barrett Esophagus

After many decades of experience with laparoscopic Heller myotomy with fundoplication, the development of Barrett esophagus has been well documented at a rate estimated between 2.5% and 6% depending on follow-up duration and protocols.[49,50] However, the rate of Barrett esophagus has been consistently higher in studies where most patients underwent myotomy alone. In an early report of open myotomy where only 4% had a concomitant fundoplication, the rate of Barrett esophagus was estimated at 6.5% at 15 years of follow-up.[51] In a pilot randomized study comparing Heller myotomy alone with Heller myotomy with a floppy Nissen, Falkenback and colleagues[52] found a rate of Barrett esophagus as high as 20% with myotomy alone.

Although these studies have several limitations, including nonstandardized follow-up, lack of information about PPI use, and retrospective nature, one can only expect that Barrett esophagus may become a significant problem in this patient population. As more and more POEM procedures are being performed worldwide, and because of its high rates of clinically silent reflux and lack of data guiding standardized follow-up protocols, it is plausible that a significant proportion of patients treated with POEM may end up with Barrett esophagus and esophageal adenocarcinoma 20 to 30 years down the road. According to current data of approximately 10 years of follow-up, the risk is considered minimal,[53] but reports of Barrett esophagus and esophageal adenocarcinoma have been reported.[54] Furthermore, the lack of standardized protocol and the fact that most reflux after POEM is clinically silent make this complication likely to be underreported. Very-long-term follow-up studies with rigorous and standardized surveillance protocols done by pioneers in the field will be useful to guide surveillance with evidence.

SUMMARY

In conclusion, perioperative complications are very uncommon if operative principles are well followed with the intent of preventing complications. Most intraoperative complications are generally managed successfully with simple endoscopic maneuvers. Although data on the occurrence of GERD after POEM are helpful, significant knowledge gaps remain regarding its prevention and its long-term consequences, such as Barrett esophagus. It is hoped this will become better defined as the technique is widely adopted and as very-long-term data are published.

CLINICS CARE POINTS

- Most intraoperative complications during per oral endoscopic myotomy are best prevented but can be managed with advanced endoscopic skills when they occur. They rarely translate into morbidity.

- Early postoperative complications, such as perforation from mucosotomy failure or intramural hematoma, are rare but translate into significant morbidity for the patient. These are almost always successfully managed endoscopically.

- The differential diagnosis of early recurrent dysphagia after per oral endoscopic myotomy includes incomplete myotomy, reflux-related stricture, excessive scarring, or incorrect initial diagnosis.

- Risk factors for post–per oral endoscopic myotomy reflux are patient-related (high body mass index, normal esophageal diameter, female gender, and lower esophageal sphincter pressure <45 mm Hg on preoperative manometry) and procedure-related (long myotomy, full-thickness myotomy, posterior myotomy, nonpreservation of the sling fibers). Up to 25% of patients with clinically significant gastroesophageal reflux disease on pH study will be asymptomatic. Most patients with reflux are well controlled with proton-pump inhibitors.

- Post–per oral endoscopic myotomy pseudodiverticulum, defined as a wide diverticulum (>2 cm) or luminal dilatation greater than 50% of the remaining esophagus at the site of the myotomy, is associated with worse quality of life and failure rates. Treatment options include laparoscopic diverticulectomy, ensuring a complete myotomy distally, or esophagectomy.

- Barrett esophagus is a well-defined problem after Heller myotomy. Although rates are considered low after per oral endoscopic myotomy, longer-term studies are needed to further define this complication after per oral endoscopic myotomy.

DISCLOSURE

F. Khazoom: None. B.E. Louie: Consultant, Implantica; Data and Safety Monitoring Board: Omega Cuff, Aplos Medical.

REFERENCES

1. Inoue H, Minami H, Kobayashi Y, et al. Peroral endoscopic myotomy (POEM) for esophageal achalasia. Endoscopy 2010;42(4):265–71.

2. Werner YB, Hakanson B, Martinek J, et al. Endoscopic or surgical myotomy in patients with idiopathic achalasia. N Engl J Med 2019;381(23):2219–29.

3. Ponds FA, Fockens P, Lei A, et al. Effect of peroral endoscopic myotomy vs pneumatic dilation on symptom severity and treatment outcomes among treatment-naive patients with achalasia: a randomized clinical trial. JAMA 2019;322(2):134–44.

4. Wang Y, Liu ZQ, Xu MD, et al. Clinical and endoscopic predictors for intraprocedural mucosal injury during per-oral endoscopic myotomy. Gastrointest Endosc 2019;89(4):769–78.

5. Axtell AL, Gaissert HA, Morse CR, et al. Management and outcomes of esophageal perforation. Dis Esophagus 2022;35(1).

6. Fujiyoshi Y, Inoue H, Abad MRA, et al. Importance of second-look endoscopy after per-oral endoscopic myotomy for safe postoperative management. Dig Endosc 2021;33(3):364–72.

7. Nabi Z, Reddy DN, Ramchandani M. Adverse events during and after per-oral endoscopic myotomy: prevention, diagnosis, and management. Gastrointest Endosc 2018;87(1):4–17.

8. Louie BE. Per oral endoscopic myotomy: technique and tricks for challenging anatomy. Operat Tech Thorac Cardiovasc Surg 2024. https://doi.org/10.1053/j.optechstcvs.2023.12.001.

9. Kurian AA, Bhayani NH, Reavis K, et al. Endoscopic suture repair of full-thickness esophagotomy during per-oral esophageal myotomy for achalasia. Surg Endosc 2013;27(10):3910.

10. Pescarus R, Shlomovitz E, Sharata AM, et al. Endoscopic suturing versus endoscopic clip closure of the mucosotomy during a per-oral endoscopic myotomy (POEM): a case-control study. Surg Endosc 2016;30(5):2132–5.

11. Zhang WG, Linghu EQ, Li HK. Fibrin sealant for closure of mucosal penetration at the cardia during peroral endoscopic myotomy: A retrospective study at a single center. World J Gastroenterol 2017;23(9):1637–44.

12. Li H, Linghu E, Wang X. Fibrin sealant for closure of mucosal penetration at the cardia during peroral endoscopic myotomy (POEM). Endoscopy 2012;44(SUPPL. 2).

13. Haito-Chavez Y, Inoue H, Beard KW, et al. Comprehensive analysis of adverse events associated with per oral endoscopic myotomy in 1826 patients: an international multicenter study. Am J Gastroenterol 2017;112(8):1267–76.

14. Drexel S, Bingmer K, Anderson M, et al. An evaluation of the complication risks following peroral endoscopic myotomy in patients on antithrombotic therapy. Surg Endosc 2021;35(10):5620–5.

15. Bechara R, Onimaru M, Ikeda H, et al. Per-oral endoscopic myotomy, 1000 cases later: pearls, pitfalls,

and practical considerations. Gastrointest Endosc 2016;84(2):330–8.

16. Pannu D, Yang D, Abbitt PL, et al. Prospective evaluation of CT esophagram findings after peroral endoscopic myotomy. Gastrointest Endosc 2016; 84(3):408–15.

17. Ichkhanian Y, Abimansour JP, Pioche M, et al. Outcomes of anterior versus posterior peroral endoscopic myotomy 2 years post-procedure: Prospective follow-up results from a randomized clinical trial. Endoscopy 2021;53(5):462–8.

18. Maher SZ, Chintanaboina J, Kim DE, et al. Pneumopericardium complicating per-oral endoscopic myotomy due to inadvertent use of air instead of carbon dioxide. ACG Case Rep J 2018;5(1):e59.

19. Banks-Venegoni AL, Desilets DJ, Romanelli JR, et al. Tension capnopericardium and cardiac arrest as an unexpected adverse event of peroral endoscopic myotomy (with video). Gastrointest Endosc 2015; 82(6):1137–9.

20. Wang L, Liu ZQ, Zhang JY, et al. Management of delayed bleeding of upper gastrointestinal endoscopic submucosal tunneling procedures: a retrospective single-center analysis and brief meta-analysis. J Gastroenterol Hepatol 2023;38(12):2174–84.

21. Zhang XC, Li QL, Xu MD, et al. Major perioperative adverse events of peroral endoscopic myotomy: a systematic 5-year analysis. Endoscopy 2016;48(11): 967–78.

22. Werner YB, von Renteln D, Noder T, et al. Early adverse events of per-oral endoscopic myotomy. Gastrointest Endosc 2017;85(4):708–18.e2.

23. Zhang YQ, Yao LQ, Xu MD, et al. Early diagnosis and management of esophageal leakage after peroral endoscopic myotomy for achalasia. Turk J Gastroenterol 2016;27(2):97–102.

24. Daza Castro EM, Fuentes CF, Córdoba Guzmán AC, et al. Multimodal endoscopic management of esophageal perforations as a complication of peroral endoscopic myotomy for a zenker's diverticulum. ACG Case Rep J 2023;10(6):e01059.

25. Smith KE, Saad AR, Hanna JP, et al. Revisional surgery in patients with recurrent dysphagia after heller myotomy. J Gastrointest Surg 2020;24(5):991–9.

26. Knight W, Kandiah K, Vrakopoulou Z, et al. Early outcomes following EndoFLIP-tailored peroral endoscopic myotomy (POEM): the establishment of POEM services in two UK centers. Dis Esophagus 2023;36(8).

27. Knowles TB, Jackson AS, Chang SC, et al. Changes in Distensibility Index During an Incremental POEM Myotomy. J Gastrointest Surg 2022;26(6):1140–6.

28. Nabi Z, Ramchandani M, Kotla R, et al. Gastroesophageal reflux disease after peroral endoscopic myotomy is unpredictable, but responsive to proton pump inhibitor therapy: A large, single-center study. Endoscopy 2020;52(8):643–51.

29. Fernandez-Ananin S, Fernández AF, Balagué C, et al. What to do when Heller's myotomy fails? Pneumatic dilatation, laparoscopic remyotomy or peroral endoscopic myotomy: A systematic review. J Minimal Access Surg 2018;14(3):177–84.

30. van Hoeij FB, Ponds FA, Werner Y, et al. Management of recurrent symptoms after per-oral endoscopic myotomy in achalasia. Gastrointest Endosc 2018;87(1):95–101.

31. Werner YB, Costamagna G, Swanström LL, et al. Clinical response to peroral endoscopic myotomy in patients with idiopathic achalasia at a minimum follow-up of 2 years. Gut 2016;65(6):899–906.

32. Tyberg A, Seewald S, Sharaiha RZ, et al. A multicenter international registry of redo per-oral endoscopic myotomy (POEM) after failed POEM. Gastrointest Endosc 2017;85(6):1208–11.

33. Wang L, Li YM. Recurrent achalasia treated with Heller myotomy: a review of the literature. World J Gastroenterol 2008;14(46):7122–6.

34. Giulini L, Dubecz A, Stein HJ. Laparoskopische Heller-Myotomie nach erfolgloser POEM und multiplen Ballondilatationen: Besser spät als nie. Chirurg 2017;88(4):303–6.

35. Jones EL, Meara MP, Schwartz JS, et al. Gastroesophageal reflux symptoms do not correlate with objective pH testing after peroral endoscopic myotomy. Surg Endosc 2016;30(3):947–52.

36. Kumbhari V, Familiari P, Bjerregaard NC, et al. Gastroesophageal reflux after peroral endoscopic myotomy: A multicenter case-control study. Endoscopy 2017;49(7):634–42.

37. Shiwaku H, Inoue H, Sasaki T, et al. A prospective analysis of GERD after POEM on anterior myotomy. Surg Endosc 2016;30(6):2496–504.

38. Rassoul Abu-Nuwar M, Eriksson SE, Sarici IS, et al. GERD after Peroral Endoscopic Myotomy: Assessment of Incidence and Predisposing Factors. J Am Coll Surg 2023;236(1):58–70.

39. Gu L, Ouyang Z, Lv L, et al. Safety and efficacy of peroral endoscopic myotomy with standard myotomy versus short myotomy for treatment-naïve patients with type II achalasia: a prospective randomized trial. Gastrointest Endosc 2021;93(6):1304–12.

40. Ramchandani M, Nabi Z, Reddy D, et al. Outcomes of anterior myotomy versus posterior myotomy during POEM: a randomized pilot study. Endosc Int Open 2018;06(02):E190–8.

41. Khashab MA, Sanaei O, Rivory J, et al. Peroral endoscopic myotomy: anterior versus posterior approach: a randomized single-blinded clinical trial. Gastrointest Endosc 2020;91(2):288–97.e7.

42. Wang XH, Tan YY, Zhu HY, et al. Full-thickness myotomy is associated with higher rate of postoperative gastroesophageal reflux disease. World J Gastroenterol 2016;22(42):9419–26.

43. Li QL, Chen WF, Zhou PH, et al. Peroral endoscopic myotomy for the treatment of achalasia: a clinical

comparative study of endoscopic full-thickness and circular muscle myotomy. J Am Coll Surg 2013; 217(3):442–51.

44. Shiwaku H, Inoue H, Shiwaku A, et al. Safety and effectiveness of sling fiber preservation POEM to reduce severe post-procedural erosive esophagitis. Surg Endosc 2022;36(6):4255–64.

45. Triggs JR, Krause AJ, Carlson DA, et al. Blown-out myotomy: an adverse event of laparoscopic Heller myotomy and peroral endoscopic myotomy for achalasia. Gastrointest Endosc 2021;93(4):861–8. e1.

46. Halder S, Acharya S, Kou W, et al. Myotomy technique and esophageal contractility impact blown-out myotomy formation in achalasia: an in silico investigation. Am J Physiol Gastrointest Liver Physiol 2022;322(5):G500–12.

47. Khan MA, Kumbhari V, Ngamruengphong S, et al. Is POEM the answer for management of spastic esophageal disorders? a systematic review and meta-analysis. Dig Dis Sci 2017;62(1):35–44.

48. Nastos D, Chen LQ, Ferraro P, et al. Long myotomy with antireflux repair for esophageal spastic disorders. J Gastrointest Surg 2002;6(5):713–22.

49. Csendes A, Orellana O, Figueroa M, et al. Long-term (17 years) subjective and objective evaluation of the durability of laparoscopic Heller esophagomyotomy in patients with achalasia of the esophagus (90% of follow-up): a real challenge to POEM. Surg Endosc 2022;36(1):282–91.

50. Jaakkola A, Reinikainen P, Ovaska J, et al. Barrett's esophagus after cardiomyotomy for esophageal achalasia. Am J Gastroenterol 1994;89(2):165–9.

51. Shai SE, Chen CY, Hsu CP, et al. Transthoracic oesophagomyotomy in the treatment of achalasia–a 15-year experience. Scand Cardiovasc J 1999;33(6): 333–6.

52. Falkenback D, Johansson J, Oberg S, et al. Heller's esophagomyotomy with or without a 360 degrees floppy Nissen fundoplication for achalasia. Long-term results from a prospective randomized study. Dis Esophagus 2003;16(4):284–90.

53. Vespa E, Pellegatta G, Chandrasekar VT, et al. Long-term outcomes of peroral endoscopic myotomy for achalasia: a systematic review and meta-analysis. Endoscopy 2023;55(2):167–75.

54. Teitelbaum EN, Dunst CM, Reavis KM, et al. Clinical outcomes five years after POEM for treatment of primary esophageal motility disorders. Surg Endosc 2018;32(1):421–7.

Complications After Paraesophageal Hernia Repair

Julie M. Corbett, MD[a], Sven E. Eriksson, MD[a,b], Inanc Samil Sarici, MD[a,b],
Blair A. Jobe, MD[a,b,c], Shahin Ayazi, MD[a,b,c,d],*

KEYWORDS

- Paraesophageal hernia • Complication • Hernia • Gastroparesis • Reherniation • Perforation
- Outcome

KEY POINTS

- Paraesophageal hernia repair (PEHR) is a technically complex operation with a challenging patient population, resulting in high morbidity and mortality due to general peri- and preoperative complications, foregut-specific complications, among others.
- Acute perioperative reherniation is rare and often asymptomatic but should be promptly repaired to minimize further complications. By contrast, early and late reherniation is common and only requires reoperation based on symptoms and anatomy.
- Use of mesh may improve early reherniation rates, but not late reherniation. Mesh-related complications are rare but can be highly morbid and increase the likelihood of organ resection.
- Perforations detected and repaired during the index operation are associated far less morbidity and mortality than those detected shortly after leaving the operating room. The longer the delay in detection, the worse the outcome.
- Gastric emptying is often delayed in the first months after PEHR, but frequently resolves spontaneously. Testing and treatment for gastroparesis should be reserved for patients with persistent symptoms.

INTRODUCTION

Paraesophageal hernia (PEH) was first described by Henry Bowditch in his *A Treatise on Diaphragmatic Hernia* in 1853.[1] At the time, PEH was thought to be an exceedingly rare condition. More than 65 years would pass before Angelo Soresi described the first hiatal hernia (HH) repair in 1919.[2] Nearly another 50 years would pass before there was sufficient experience to develop data-driven recommendations for paraesophageal hernia repair (PEHR). Skinner and Belsey published one of the most influential early papers on PEHR

outcomes in 1967.[3] They studied a cohort of 1030 HH, including 87 PEH. They initially managed 21 patients with asymptomatic PEH medically, but 6 patients died of acute PEH-related complications. These results ushered in the first era of ubiquitous asymptomatic PEHR. The rationale for elective repair of PEH irrespective of symptoms was that the morbidity and mortality of emergent PEHR was substantially higher than elective repair.

The somewhat controversial ubiquitous PEHR approach was widely adopted and remained prevalent until 2002 when Stylopoulos and Rattner published their Markov decision analytic model

[a] Foregut Division, Surgical Institute, Allegheny Health Network, 4815 Liberty Avenue, Suite 454, Pittsburgh, PA 15224, USA; [b] Chevalier Jackson Research Foundation, Esophageal Institute, Western Pennsylvania Hospital, Pittsburgh, PA, USA; [c] Department of Surgery, Drexel University, Philadelphia, PA, USA; [d] 4815 Liberty Avenue, Suite 454, Pittsburgh, PA 15224, USA
* Corresponding author.4815 Liberty Avenue, Suite 454, Pittsburgh, PA 15224.
E-mail address: shahin.ayazi@gmail.com

Thorac Surg Clin 34 (2024) 355–369
https://doi.org/10.1016/j.thorsurg.2024.06.002
1547-4127/24/© 2024 Elsevier Inc. All rights reserved, including those for text and data mining, AI training, and similar technologies.

comparing the quality-adjusted life-years benefit of observation versus elective repair for asymptomatic PEH.[4] They found that watchful waiting was the optimal treatment strategy in 83% of patients, which induced a paradigm shift in PEH management and marked the start of the asymptomatic observation era. However, Stylopoulos and colleagues acknowledged that their data was limited to mortality rates of open transabdominal or transthoracic operations. Observation would no longer be recommended in their model if elective mortality dropped below 0.5%.

From 2000 to 2013, the percent of PEH performed laparoscopically increased from 4.9% to 91.4%, changing the landscape of PEHR outcomes.[5] Recently DeMeester and colleagues published a similar Markov model with the updated laparoscopic data, using data suggesting the age-based elective PEHR morality rate ranges from 0.2% to 1.8%, below the old model's 0.5% threshold.[6] The new model demonstrated that elective PEHR is the preferred strategy for 100% of 10000 simulations at age 65, 98% at 80, 90% at 85, and 59% in a women aged 90 years. We anticipate that this study will usher in the second era of ubiquitous asymptomatic PEHR (**Fig. 1**).

At the cusp of this paradigm shift, which will likely increase the utilization of surgery in the management of PEH, it is imperative to understand the complications of PEHR. Patients who undergo PEH repair suffer more complications than those who undergo sliding HH repair as part of their antireflux surgery. They tend to be older with more comorbidities and the surgical repair of PEH is technically more challenging than HH. A National Surgical Quality Improvement Program (NSQIP) database study showed that compared to gastroesophageal reflux disease patients, PEH patients had significantly higher mortality (0.85% vs 0.18%, $P=.003$), were more likely to receive intraoperative blood transfusion (3.26% vs 0.58%, $P = .001$), and were more likely to require reoperation (4.03% vs 1.26%, $P = .001$).[7] This article will review the data on different types of complications of PEHR with a focus on recognition, etiology, and management.

OVERALL PREVALENCE AND CONTRIBUTING FACTORS

Risk assessment of PEHR complications requires careful consideration of complication-specific factors. However, there is also value in considering all cause morbidity and mortality after PEHR. Studies estimate the risk of any complication after PEHR to range between 6.6% and 38%, reoperation risk between 3% and 4.9%, and mortality between

0.37% and 2.7%.[8–16] The largest single-center study reporting their experience with PEHR from 1997 to 2008 in 662 patients reported 19% overall major morbidity, with complications rates including 4% pneumonia, 2.6% congestive heart failure, 3.4% pulmonary embolism (PE), 2.5% postoperative leak, 0.8% perioperative hernia recurrence, 2.6% need for re-intubation, 0.9% acute renal failure, 0.6% cerebrovascular accident, and 0.9% myocardial infarction. They also reported an 8% readmission rate, a 4.9% need for reoperation, and a 1.7% mortality rate.[9] These data are consistent with another study that included patients with up to 20-year follow-up. They reported 8% overall morbidity, 0.9% 30-day mortality, and a reoperation rate of 4.8%.[10] Pooled data from a systematic review and meta-analysis comprising 4428 PEHRs indicate a 16% overall complication rate, with 5% considered major complications. Reoperation was required by 4% and mortality was 1.4%.[11] Collectively, these studies suggest that PEHR is a morbid procedure with substantial mortality. However, it is important to consider factors such as urgency of the operation, surgical technique, PEH size, patient factors, and specific types of complications during a tailored risk assessment.

Studies assessing risk factors for all-cause morbidity and mortality have found that urgent versus elective repair is among the most impactful factors (**Table 1**). One study found a 7.5% mortality rate for urgent repair, compared to only 0.5% for elective.[9] A similar study from the same center including 980 patients found that urgency of PEHR was a predictor of both major morbidity (41% vs 18%, $P<.001$) and mortality (8% vs 1%, $P<.001$).[12] Another study from this center found that emergent repair was more likely to result in major complications (38% vs 18%, $P<.001$), including pulmonary complications, myocardial infarction, congestive heart failure, atrial fibrillation, *Clostridium* difficile infection, delirium, and acute renal insufficiency. Additionally urgent PEHR was associated with prolonged ventilation, re-intubation, and blood transfusion, contributing to a longer length of stay.[13]

The benefits of laparoscopic surgery over open surgery are clear for many procedures, including PEHR. Compared to open, studies report that laparoscopic PEHR results in lower blood loss, fewer intraoperative complications, quicker return to normal diet, reduced opioid requirements, and shorter hospital length of stay, with comparable results on general and disease specific quality of life measures.[14,15] Other factors, such as larger PEH size are associated with more intraoperative complications, postoperative complications and

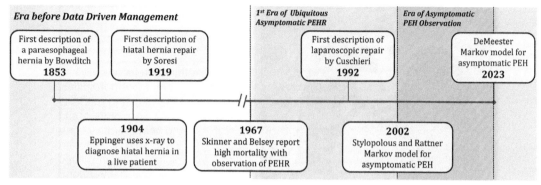

Fig. 1. Key events in the timeline of the paraesophageal hernia repair.

a higher comprehensive complication index (CCI) score.[16] Age greater than or equal to 70 and CCI greater than or equal to 3 have also been associated with a 67% increased risk of major nonfatal adverse outcome (**Table 1**).[9] In a large single center study, they developed predictive models suggesting that age greater than 80, urgency of operation, congestive heart failure, and pulmonary disease were covariate risk factors for postoperative mortality. These same factors plus male sex and decades of life over 50 were predictors of overall morbidity.[12]

REHERNIATION

Reherniation can be a distressing and confusing complication for patients. The literature supports a pragmatic approach, focusing on whether the patient is symptomatic and whether the risks of watchful waiting outweigh revisional surgery, to determine whether reherniation is a concerning finding. Reherniation can be broadly categorized into 3 groups based on onset or detection: acute perioperative, early, and late.

Acute Perioperative Reherniation

Acute perioperative reherniation after PEHR is rare. As a result of heterogeneity in the definition of 'acute' (7–30 days from index operation), the incidence of acute perioperative reherniation has a reported range of 0.8% to 2.8%.[9,17,18] There is a paucity of the data on risk factors for acute perioperative reherniation. However, one study suggested that size of the defect has a stepwise relationship with incidence of reherniation, reporting 5.3%

Table 1
Risk factors for paraesophageal hernia repair complications supported by literature

Complication	Incidence	Risk Factors
Any complication	6.6%–38%	Urgent repair Size of the defect Comprehensive complication index Age
Acute reherniation	0.8%–2.8%	Size of the defect
Early/Late reherniation	15%–57%	Time since surgery Spinal deformities
Gastroparesis	4.4%–18.6%	Revisional PEHR Anterior and posterior sutures Excision of the hernia sac Division of the short gastric vessels Type II PEH Diabetes
Perforation	1%–3%	BMI $\geq$35 Revisional PEHR Collis gastroplasty

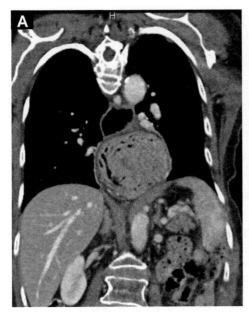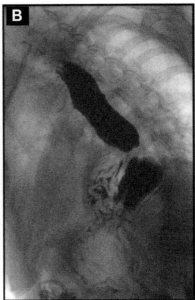

Fig. 2. Thoracoabdominal CT and barium esophagram showing a patient with late recurrence after PEHR. (*A*) Coronal contrast-enhanced CT image demonstrates a large recurrent PEH. (*B*) Barium swallow study shows large paraesophageal hernia with poor barium clearance and dilated esophagus. CT, Computerized tomography; PEHR, Paraesophageal hernia repair; PEH, Paraesophageal hernia.

incidence in patients with an intra-thoracic stomach, 2.7% with greater than 5 cm defect and 1.4% with less than 5 cm defect (*P* = .001).[17]

Recognition of acute perioperative reherniation can be a challenge, as one study reported that 88.2% of 17 patients with radiographic reherniation within 7 days of index operation were asymptomatic.[18] Other studies have similarly reported that the vast majority of acute perioperative reherniations are clinically silent.[17] These studies argue empiric esophagram is warranted. But, given the low incidence of acute reherniation requiring reoperation some have questioned the necessity of esophagram. However, other studies have suggested that empiric postoperative esophagram reduces the morbidity associated with reoperation. One study of 1571 patients with HH (50.4% PEH) who underwent routine esophagram and 258 patients (49.6% PEH) without esophagram, found immediate reherniation was detected in 1.5% of patients with esophagram, 87.5% of which underwent reoperation. Of patients without esophagram, 0.8% underwent reoperation for symptoms. When they compared the impact of esophagram on outcome of early reoperation, they found that use of esophagram was associated with a shorter time between index operation and reoperation (2.4 vs 4.3 days, *P* = .037) and a lower morbidity (13.5 vs 85.7%, *P*<.001) and mortality rate (0.0 vs 14.3%, *P* = .16).[17] These findings highlight the

benefits of earlier recognition. This study also compared outcomes of early reoperation to reoperation for late reherniation, which similarly found that early reoperation was associated with fewer intraoperative and postoperative complications. Additionally, at 1 year follow-up, early reoperation patients had less dysphagia to solids and greater satisfaction with their hernia repair.

Early and Late Reherniation

After the perioperative period, reherniation has been broadly further subdivided into early reherniation (before 6-month), and late reherniation (after 6-month) (**Fig. 2**). However, the majority of the literature that makes this temporal distinction focus on mesh and reherniation. There are 2 randomized control trials (RCTs) that found mesh results in significantly lower rates of reherniation than suture cruroplasty at 6-month. However, both studies demonstrate that after 6-month this benefit disappears.[19,20] The remainder of the literature on non-acute perioperative reherniation does not make any meaningful distinction between early and late.

The rate of early or late reherniations in the literature ranges between 5% and 57%. This variability is likely due to heterogeneity regarding size of PEH, surgical technique and follow-up. Generally, over longer follow-up periods the reherniation rate increases, with studies exceeding 50% reherniation after 5 years.[20,21] One study of 146 patients who underwent PEHR with annual empiric esophagrams found that there was a stepwise increase in the prevalence of reherniation each year from less than 5% at 1 year to greater than 25% at 3 years.[22] This is consistent with a study, which followed 455 patients for up to 20 years that found the cumulative reherniation rate to be 13.7% within 1 year, 30.8% within 5 years, 40.1% within 10 years, and 50.0% after 10 years.[10] Surgeon experience also impacts reherniation rates. A study comparing PEHR outcomes performed via laparotomy (n = 13), thoracotomy (n = 14), and laparoscopy (n = 27) from 1985 to 1998, found that reherniation occurred in 42% of laparoscopic cases, but only 15% of open (P<.001).[23] However, the same group published their data from 1998 to 2010, comprising 73 laparoscopic and 73 open PEHRs, and found the results flipped, with fewer reherniations after laparoscopic PEHR (12.3% vs 24.7%, P = .09).[22] These studies suggest that as the authors' laparoscopic experience improved so did their rates of reherniation. Requisite experience with this technically complex operation and its associated complication rate may be responsible for a spontaneous centralization of PEHR practice to high-volume centers. A National Inpatient Sample database study assessing PEHRs performed per 100 patients between 2000 and 2011 found that PEHR significantly increased from 65.8 to 94.4 at high-volume hospitals, but the number of procedures at low- and intermediate-volume hospitals has decreased from 9.0 and 25.2 to 1.2 and 4.4, respectively. All cause complications were also much lower at high volume institutions (12.7% vs 26.4% and 24.1%, respectively, P<.0001).[24]

The majority of patients who undergo PEHR receive a fundoplication to aid in the prevention of reherniation and control reflux. Magnetic sphincter augmentation (MSA) has proven to be a similarly effective procedure in terms of reflux control. However, limited data suggest that MSA may also be effective with PEHR. One study of 22 patients who underwent PEHR with MSA found 20% reherniation rate 1 year after surgery (Fig. 3). Additionally, outcomes were similar between PEH and large and small HH.[25] By contrast, another study of 200 patients, 78% of which had greater than or equal to 5 cm HH or PEH, who underwent MSA, reported no reherniations.[26] These data must be interpreted in context of the selection criteria for MSA. To mitigate complications from the physiologic challenge of MSA, patients routinely undergo a complete preoperative esophageal physiology workup to select patients with good esophageal motility. Studies have suggested that poor esophageal motility is more common in patients with PEH.[27] Therefore, MSA data only represent a selection of patients with good motility despite PEH and cannot necessarily be extrapolated to the larger PEH population, who commonly undergo an abbreviated workup or require unplanned urgent or emergent PEHR, with no exclusion of patients with poor esophageal motility.

Some studies have suggested that the timing of reherniation is related to its etiology. One study looked at 108 consecutive patients with reherniation following a posterior PEHR. They found that the majority of reherniations were anterior defects stretching to the left of the esophagus (67%), followed by circumferential defects (21%) and posterior defects (12%). Time to reherniation for anterior defects (3.5 years) was significantly longer than for posterior defects (1.5 years), suggesting that earlier reherniation was due to breakdown of the primary repair, while later reherniation was due to chronic and repeated stress eventually overcoming the tensile strength of the hiatus.[28]

The reherniation rate may be high, but fortunately multiple studies have demonstrated most are asymptomatic and rarely need reoperation.[18,21,29] One study reporting a 30% reherniation rate at 45 months after PEHR, found that 89% of reherniations were asymptomatic.[30] Long-term studies with high rates of reherniation have shown similar results. One study followed 108 patients for up to 7 years and found that, despite reherniation increasing from 14% at 6 months to 57% at final follow-up, only 2 patients (3%) developed symptoms requiring reoperation.[20] Another study found that reherniation made no difference to quality of life measures up to 20 years after PEHR.[10] These studies support observation for the majority asymptomatic reherniations.

There are limited data that development symptomatic reherniation may be related to the postoperative HH-type anatomy. One study reported that of their 11 patients with reherniation, 4 were asymptomatic, with postoperative Type I HH anatomy more likely to be asymptomatic than Type II or III (100% vs 12.5%, P<.05).[21] This study indicated that symptoms should potentially increase the index of suspicion for a PEH reherniation. Collectively, these studies suggest observation for asymptomatic reherniation may be appropriate for most patients, while symptomatic reherniation should be repaired.

Limited studies have attempted to identify risk factors for reherniation and need for reoperation. A study of 70 PEHRs found that at 4 years, 89% of patients were asymptomatic and 70% of repairs were intact. Age, sex, body mass index (BMI), PEH

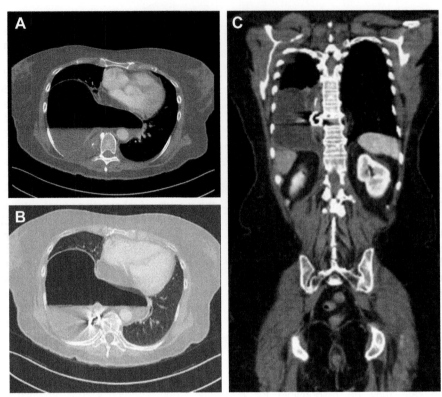

Fig. 3. Postoperative thoracoabdominal CT images showing acute re-herniation after use of MSA with PEHR. (*A*) Axial chest CT image showing dilated stomach and severe esophageal angulation suggesting possible gastric volvulus. (*B*) Axial chest CT image showing dilated stomach with MSA implant herniated to the right chest. (*C*) Coronal thoracoabdominal CT image showing the herniation of the stomach and MSA implant to the right chest with suspected gastric volvulus. CT, Computerized tomography; MSA, Magnetic sphincter augmentation, PEHR, Paraesophageal hernia repair.

type, addition of fundoplication, and duration of follow-up were not predictors of reherniation or symptoms.[30] A prospective study of 70 patients who underwent PEHR similarly found that no clinical factors were associated with recurrence, including age, sex, BMI, smoking status, diabetes mellitus, pulmonary disease, previous abdominal surgery, preoperative dysphagia, heartburn, or pain.[18] One study of 662 patients who underwent giant PEH repair similarly found that the majority of clinical characteristics were not factors.[9]

There is only population of patients, which clearly do have an elevated risk of reherniation: those with spinal deformities. A study comparing PEHR outcomes between 86 patients with spinal deformities (kyphosis, lordosis, and scoliosis) to 460 patients without spinal deformities found that deformities were associated with higher recurrence rate (47.7% vs 30.0%, $P = .001$), shorter time to recurrence (10.3 vs 19.2 months, $P = .02$), and larger recurrence (5 vs 4 cm, $P = .01$).[31] Apart from spinal deformity, these studies provide limited clinical information to predict

postoperative reherniation or need for reoperation. If a patient remains asymptomatic outside of the perioperative period, an esophagram is unlikely to alter management, but symptomatic patients should be evaluated for recurrence and repaired.

Mesh-related Complications

Most PEHR reports implement primary sutured crural repair. However, due to the high reherniation rate some have suggested mesh reinforcement may increase PEHR resilience to stress and prevent reherniation. While biologic mesh has long been thought of as a safer alternative to synthetic, it has not been proven effective for long-term prevention of reherniation. Mesh cruroplasty remains controversial due to concerns over its long-term efficacy, complications (eg, erosion, dysphagia, and stricture formation), and its impact on the technical feasibility of revisional surgery. As a result, there has been a trend away from the utilization of mesh. An NSQIP database study of 25801 PEHRs found that mesh utilization dropped from 46.2% to 35.2% (P<.001) between 2010 and 2017.[32]

There have been limited reports of devastating complications due to mesh. The most alarming study is a multicenter case-series of 28 patients who had mesh complications requiring reoperation. These included: dysphagia (n = 22), heartburn (n = 10), chest pain (n = 14), fever (n = 1), epigastric pain (n = 2), and weight loss (n = 4), which were due to mesh erosion (n = 17), esophageal stenosis (n = 6), and dense fibrosis (n = 5). Esophagectomy was required in 21%. Type of mesh or repair had no impact on complications.[33] This study suggests that mesh is associated with devastating outcomes. However, because this was a multicenter case-series, specifically gathering data on mesh-related complications, there is no information to provide an assessment of incidence or relative risk of these complications. Nevertheless, other studies have also linked mesh to higher rates of esophagectomy. A single center case series of 26 patients who had revisional PEHR after mesh found that esophagectomy was required in 27% of cases and 22% required a Roux-en Y gastrojejunostomy. The most frequent presenting symptom was dysphagia (56%) with mesh erosion in 12% of patients.[34] The reason for the increased need for resection is the increased complexity of the anatomy with mesh in place. A study comparing 10 mesh revisions to 68 non-mesh revisional PEHRs found that mesh was associated with a reduced ability to create a fundoplication (20% vs 62%, P = .03) and a 6.8-fold increased risk of requiring a major resection (P = .05).[35] These studies demonstrate that there is substantial risk of complicated and technically difficult revisional surgery with the use of mesh. However, data on the incidence of these complications are limited, and studies not specifically focused on revisional surgery have demonstrated no adverse mesh-related outcomes, suggesting the incidence may be low. Two RCTs and an NSQIP study found that there was no association between mesh and increased complications.[19,20,32] The most robust assessment of the risk of mesh complications available comes from a systematic review and meta-analysis, which found that among 4000 pooled patients, the incidence of mesh complications was 1.8%, with mesh-erosion affecting only 0.035% of patients. They also found that synthetic mesh was more frequently associated with erosion requiring intervention than biologic mesh.[36] Large multicenter studies are necessary to determine the greater impact of mesh-related complications; however, multiple small studies suggest that this is a potentially devastating, yet rare complication.

Gastroparesis

Preservation of the vagal innervation during extensive mediastinal dissection in the setting of distorted PEH anatomy is a challenge, putting patients at risk for post-surgical gastroparesis. Studies have demonstrated gastroparesis after PEHR has a detrimental impact on patient satisfaction, with some reporting nearly 20% of patients with post-surgical gastroparesis regret the decision to undergo surgery.[37] If these bothersome nausea, vomiting, bloating, early satiety, and weight loss symptoms persist, an additional procedure to treat the gastroparesis may be required. Fortunately, studies have demonstrated that a pyloric drainage surgery for post-surgical gastroparesis after PEHR can be effective, significantly improving patient's symptom scores (P = .0002) and improving 4-h gastric retention on gastric emptying scintigraphy from 46.4% to 17.9%, with 50% gastric emptying normalization.[38]

The reported incidence of postsurgical gastroparesis is highly variable due to the heterogeneous definition of gastroparesis in the literature. Studies using definitions based on 6-month endoscopic findings of retained food despite a 6-h fast have reported rates as high as 18.6%.[37] Arguably, the most representative estimate of the incidence of gastroparesis after PEHR comes from a New York State database study of 2144 patients who underwent primary PEHR over a 5 year period. They found that only 95 (4.4%) patients had either a diagnosis of gastroparesis or required surgical intervention for gastroparesis.[39] This comparatively low rate is consistent with other studies reporting that this complication occurs in less than 5% of cases.[37,40]

Gastroparesis may be relatively rare after a primary PEHR, but multiple studies have demonstrated higher rates following revisional PEHR.[37,41,42] Hamrick and colleagues reviewed the records of 284 recurrent PEHRs over an 8 years period and found that 12% of patients required an intervention for gastroparesis following a single revisional PEHR. However, among patients who required a second revisional PEHR, the rate was 66%. The rate increased to 75% for those requiring a third revisional PEHR.[42] This study suggests that gastroparesis is an expected outcome in patients requiring multiple revisional PEHRs, and should be discussed with patients during risk stratification, patient selection, and expectation management for additional revisional repairs. Another study found that revisional PEHR (OR: 6.2, P = .021) was an independent predictor of postoperative gastroparesis. They compared 19 patients with delayed gastric emptying to 83 patients without delayed emptying at 6 months following a PEHR, focusing on technical and patient risk factors associated with delayed emptying. Technical risk factors associated with delayed emptying on univariate analysis included placement of both anterior and posterior sutures for hiatal closure (63% vs 34%, $P = .035$), excision of the hernia sac from the gastric cardia (47% vs 16%, $P = .002$), division of the short gastric vessels (42% vs 10%, $P = .002$), and revisional surgery (26% vs 5%, $P = .011$). Among patient factors, they looked at age, sex, BMI, diabetes status, type of PEH, and use of proton pump inhibitors, prokinetic agents, and antikinetic agents. However, the only patient factor that was significant was presence of a type II PEH (58% vs 24%, $P = .006$). The authors argue that the common theme among risk-factors is that they involve more surgical manipulation with high-energy devices in a confined space in close proximity to the vagus nerve, promoting injury. Interestingly, diabetes was not a factor in this study.[37] However, in the aforementioned New York State database study, they found that diabetes was a strongly correlated with the diagnosis of post-surgical gastroparesis.[39] This is an expected risk factor, as diabetes has been implicated as a major cause of gastroparesis. In a patient with diabetes, it is not entirely clear whether gastroparesis is due to surgical intervention or a complication of their diabetes.

Emptying scintigraphy is the most reliable test to confirm that a patient's symptoms are due to delayed gastric emptying. However, in a patient with a PEH, the distorted anatomy and at least partially intrathoracic stomach may delay emptying or even promote food trapping, which interferes with the accuracy of the study. Therefore, there is a high risk of a false positive for delayed gastric emptying on gastric emptying scintigraphy prior to PEHR. As such there is no reliable test to determine if postoperative gastroparesis symptoms are caused by surgery or were simply revealed by restoration of normal anatomy. Additionally, timing of the gastric emptying assessment is an important factor to consider after PEHR. Transient-delayed gastric emptying has been described in patients following laparoscopic antireflux surgery. One study of 51 patients with no preoperative evidence of delayed gastric emptying found that 92.2% of patients had endoscopic evidence of delayed emptying at 1 month with associated gastroparesis-like symptoms; however, by 2 months 0% had endoscopic delayed emptying and symptoms resolved.[43] This study suggests that some degree of gastric emptying delay is expected in the early perioperative period but resolves spontaneously in most cases. Therefore,

index of suspicion for gastroparesis should remain low during the perioperative period and objective investigation should be delayed until the patients' symptoms have established themselves as persistent.

Perforation

Esophageal perforation represents one of the most potentially devastating complications of PEHR (**Fig. 4**). Studies estimate that approximately 1% to 3% of PEHR will have an iatrogenic perforation.[9,44] Both management and prognosis differ dramatically depending on whether perforation is recognized prior to leaving the operating room. Studies have demonstrated that delayed perforation is more likely to require critical care and carries an estimated mortality rate of 17%.[45] One study assessing perforation among 1223 patients found that perforations discovered postoperatively were more likely to require reoperation (75% vs 2%; $P<.001$), to require more gastrointestinal and radiologic interventions (50% vs 2%; $P=.004$), and to have higher morbidity (88% vs 26%; $P=.004$) than perforations recognized intraoperatively.[44] Therefore, it is imperative that care be taken to minimize the risk of perforation and to recognize perforation intraoperatively. Studies have found that the most common mechanism of perforation during PEHR is traction (43%) during reduction of the hernia, followed by suture placement, bougie insertion, and thermal injury.[44] The risk of a traction injury can be ameliorated by performing a complete mediastinal dissection and mobilization of the esophagus prior to attempting reduction, minimizing traction required. Fortunately, most perforations are recognized intraoperatively, with studies reporting detection of 84% of perforations before leaving the operative room.[44] Utilization of an intraoperative leak test may improve identification of a perforation prior to the completion of a PEHR. Postoperative radiographic studies can also aid in early leak detection, with studies showing up to 83% leak detection, resulting in earlier intervention and superior outcomes than those undetected.[44] Postoperative leak tests are also useful in patients with a known intraoperative perforation, with studies showing that up to 5% of patients with known repaired intraoperative perforations have persistent leak on early perioperative radiography.[44]

There are limited data on risk factors for leak. Luketich and colleagues found that the odds of postoperative leak were increased 3.8 times in patients with BMI greater than or equal to 35[9]. Another study found that 1/3rd of patients with a postoperative leak following an antireflux operation had

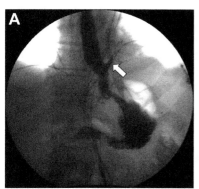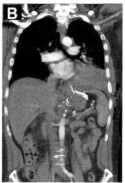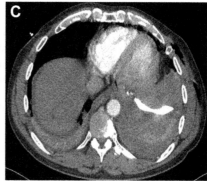

Fig. 4. Radiographic imaging of a patient with postoperative leak and hemothorax following laparoscopic PEHR (*A*) Barium esophagram showing focal extravasation of contrast (*arrow*) from the distal esophagus (*B*) Coronal chest CT image showing contrast extravasation and moderate left hemothorax. (*C*) Axial chest CT image showing the contrast extravasation and left sided hemothorax. CT, Computerized tomography, PEHR, Paraesophageal hernia repair.

undergone a previous hiatal operation.[45] Patients requiring Collis gastroplasty are another group of patients that are at increased risk of postoperative leak.[9]

When an intraoperative perforation is detected, studies have demonstrated good outcomes with either a single- or 2-layer absorbable suture repair. Fundoplication may be used to buttress the repair if location allows. A trans-hiatal drain should be placed adjacent to the repair, with the patient 'nothing by mouth' for 24 to 48 hours prior to confirmation of leak resolution. Elevated drain amylase is an indicator that the leak has not resolved. However, confirmation with a clinical leak test should be obtained prior to starting a diet. Drain placement can be beneficial if there is concern for an intraoperative leak without an obvious source. A review of 1005 foregut procedures found that patients who were diagnosed with a leak postoperatively did well with conservative management when they already had adequate drainage at the time of diagnosis.[45]

The management of perforation diagnosed after the initial surgery most frequently requires a return to the operating room. Studies have demonstrated that delay in diagnosis may be caused by attributing signs to other causes in the early postoperative period, particularly fever.[45] Once the diagnosis is confirmed, treatment should focus on minimizing contamination and repair of the perforation. Primary buttressed suture repair may be possible, depending on the size of the perforation and the friability of the tissue. Endoscopic clips are another option for some perforations. Studies have demonstrated successful closure of up to 25 mm perforations at a median of 18 days after clip application. Esophageal stents have also been successfully deployed to treat perforations with the added benefit of facilitating earlier enteral feeding. The major risk with stents is migration, reported in up to 37.5% of cases. When used for perforation, the risk of migration is thought to be slightly higher due to the absence of the narrowing that keeps the stent in place in stricture or malignancy. Another option for some perforations is endoluminal vacuum. The negative pressure and sponge provide both source control and debridement of the tissue, facilitating healing. Limited studies have reported 86% of perforations successfully resolve with the use of endoluminal vacuum therapy.[46] In severe cases, particularly in patients with poor nutritional status, those with several days of undiagnosed leak, or the presence of severely inflamed or ischemic tissue, a full diversion may be required.

PULMONARY COMPLICATIONS
Pneumothorax

During PEHR, extensive mediastinal dissection is necessary, and the distorted anatomy can make this process technically difficult and time consuming. As a result, patients are at risk of complications related to carbon dioxide insufflation, including subcutaneous emphysema, pneumothorax, pneumomediastinum, and pneumopericardium. There are no studies specifically looking at risk factors for pneumothorax in PEHR. However, studies assessing risk of pneumothorax in laparoscopy have found that HH surgery is a risk factor (odds ratio [OR]: 3.18), in addition to an end tidal carbon dioxide of 50 mm Hg or greater (OR 4.15) and an operative time more than 200 minutes (OR 20.5).[47] In large PEHR an exacerbating factor is the chronically low cardiopulmonary reserve due to herniation of abdominal contents into the thorax. The first indication that a pleural violation has occurred may be indicated by increased airway pressures, end-tidal carbon dioxide, and heart rate with decreased oxygen saturation and blood pressure intraoperatively.[48]

There is paucity of the data on the management of pneumothorax after PEHR. Early case reports advocated aggressive management with immediate desufflation and a percutaneous chest tube before continuing laparoscopically under low pressure, high flow pneumoperitoneum.[49] Experience with homeostatic derangement during esophagectomy has born the technique of placing a trans-hiatal drain laparoscopically and bringing it out through a laparoscopic port can be highly effective.[50] These remain options in principle for a patient that is unable to tolerate the homeostatic insult. However, with more experience it has become anecdotally clear that pneumothorax during laparoscopy is largely tolerated well by patients with minimal impact on outcome or perioperative symptomatology. A recent study from Swedish Medical Center reviewed 2268 cases of minimally invasive HH repair and identified pleurotomies in 16.2% of this cohort. These pleurotomies were opened widely and managed intraoperatively with changes in insufflation and anesthesia support. They found the overall rate of complications was similar in those with pleural violation to a matched group of patients with no violation (19.8% vs 21.2%, $P = .66$). The rate of pleural effusions requiring intervention was also comparable between the groups.[51]

In practice, we have found that perioperative dyspnea is rarely related to pleural violation or capnothorax (**Fig. 5**). This largely resolves during intraoperative desufflation, and any remaining carbon dioxide is absorbed and exhaled.[52] Therefore, significant perioperative dyspnea should prompt a thorough workup, as it may potentially represent a more sinister underlying cause.

Pneumonia and Effusion

The highest index of suspicion for perioperative dyspnea should be for pneumonia or pleural effusion. The presence of a large portion of the stomach in the chest chronically reduces the patient's functional lung capacity and promotes gastroesophageal reflux. This refluxogenic anatomy in conjunction with supine positioning and anesthetic suppression of airway protective reflexes puts patients at elevated risk of aspiration during anesthesia induction for PEHR. In addition, microaspirations may not be fully recognized until a postoperative pneumonia is diagnosed. An additional factor that can affect pulmonary function is reduction of a large volume of intrathoracic abdominal contents, which can lead to fluid shifts and development of pleural effusion. The risks of these complications are apparent in the literature. In Luketich and colleagues report on their 10 years' experience with giant PEHR, they found that pleural effusion (9%) and pneumonia (4%) were the most common major adverse perioperative outcomes.[9] This is consistent with studies on emergent repair. A single center review of a decade of emergency PEHR found that pneumonia was the most common perioperative complication affecting 35.1%.[53]

Pulmonary Embolism

Another common major perioperative complication reported by Luketich and colleagues may also present as dyspnea, PE. They found that 3.4% of patients developed PE in the perioperative setting.[9] A review of incidence following PEHR found that the pooled rate of PE was 0.842%, which was much higher than the incidence of PE after laparoscopic cholecystectomy, at 0.018-%.[54] This limited review suggests PEHR is associated with an elevated risk of PE compared to other laparoscopic procedures.

ADDITIONAL CONSIDERATIONS
Robotic Surgery

The introduction of robotic-assisted laparoscopic surgery into the surgeon's armamentarium has spawned debate over whether traditional laparoscopic or robotic surgery is superior for just about every conceivable abdominal surgery, and PEHR is no exception. One study assessed 517864 patients who underwent PEHR (11.3% robotic) in the Nationwide Readmission database and found that robotic repair was associated with a higher complication rate (9.2% vs 6.8%, $P<.001$) and more frequent readmissions, both 30-day (7.4 vs 6.1%, $P<.001$) and 90-day (11.2 vs 9.4%, $P<.001$). Specifically, robotic surgery was associated with significantly more infections, perforations, and respiratory, cardiac, and renal complications. The only complication where robotic surgery had a lower rate was bleeding, but it was not significant (1.7 vs 1.9%, $P = .141$).[55] A similarly designed study using the National Inpatient Sample database and 168329 patients who underwent PEHR (6% robotic) similarly found higher rates of overall adjusted complications (13.3% vs 11.3%, $P = .005$).[56] These national database studies suggest that robotic repair may be associated with worse outcomes.

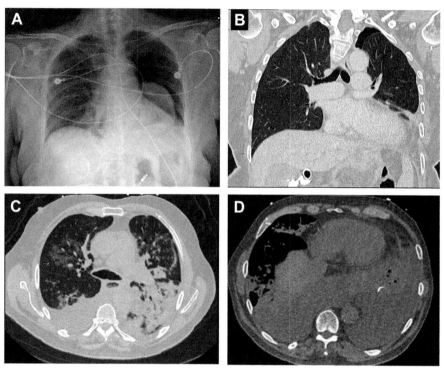

Fig. 5. Acute pulmonary complications after PEHR. (*A*) Chest X-ray with large left sided capnothorax and bilateral subcutaneous emphysema. (*B*) Coronal chest CT image showing left sided hydropneumothorax (*arrow*) following PEHR (*C*) Axial chest CT image showing multi-lobar airspace disease and bilateral pleural effusions following aspiration perioperatively for PEHR (*D*) Axial chest CT image showing large bilateral pleural effusions with compressive atelectasis. CT, Computerized tomography; PEHR, Paraesophageal hernia repair.

Limited retrospective institutional studies report contrasting results to the national database studies. One single arm study reported that 5 years after robotic PEHR only 9% of 145 patients had reherniation, which is lower than the majority of 5 years reports for laparoscopic reherniation.[57] Another study compared 278 laparoscopic repairs to 114 robotic repairs and reported no difference in complication or readmission rates. They also reported lower rates of reherniation with robotic repair (13.3 vs 32.8%, $P = .008$). However, robotic repair had a much shorter follow-up time (15 vs 24 months, $P<.001$), which, as discussed earlier, has a major impact on reherniation rates. Additionally, robotic hernias were more likely to be revisional repairs (24.5 vs 12.9%, $P = .08$).[58] Therefore, this study suggests robotic surgery may be superior, but has substantial methodologic issues. Another single-center study comparing 142 robotic to 151 repairs similarly found lower rates of complications with robotic surgery (6.3 vs 19.2%, $P = .001$).[59] However, this study also had methodologic limitations, reporting significant differences in American Society of Anesthesiologists' class, type of hernia, type of fundoplication constructed, and percent of revisional surgeries

between groups, all of which can confound differences in outcome. A systematic review and meta-analysis assessing both the outcomes and risk of bias in the literature found similar result. They compared 7 studies comprising 10078 patients and found that robotic repair was associated with fewer complications (3.5 vs 4.3%, $P = .000$). However, they determined that every study had at least a moderate "overall risk of bias" with at least a moderate 'baseline confounding' risk in their designs.[60] These studies suggest that there may be some benefit to robotic surgery, but there are no studies unmarred by substantial methodologic bias. Therefore, the additional data using more equitable and controlled groups are necessary to draw any sound conclusions regarding the relationship between PEHR complications and robotic versus traditional laparoscopic techniques.

Other Complications

There are a number of less frequently reported complications that have been described in the literature. Dysphagia is a complication of PEH that has been linked to a multitude of

Table 2
Paraesophageal hernia complications

Foregut Complications	Pulmonary Complications	Cardiovascular Complications	Other Medical Complications

Reherniation
• Acute perioperative
• Early/Late
Perforation/leak
Gastroparesis
Mesh/Pledget-related
  complications
• Erosion
• Dysphagia
• Stricture
• Dense fibrosis
Excess intestinal gas
Fistula
Gastric ischemia and
  perforation
Dysphagia
	Pneumonia
	Pleural effusion
	Pneumothorax
	Subcutaneous
	  Emphysema
	Pulmonary embolism
		Congestive heart failure
		Myocardial infarction
		Cerebrovascular accident
		Atrial fibrillation
			Renal insufficiency
			Infection
			Delirium
			Pancreatitis
			SMV thrombosis
			Splenic infarct
			Splenic injury/bleeding

complications including tight fundoplication, hiatal closure technique, angulation of the esophagus, mesh use, and reherniation, among others. Another complication that can present with dysphagia is pledget erosion. One center reported a case of a patient who presented 11 months after PEHR with severe dysphagia secondary to Teflon pledget erosion into the esophageal wall, which was able to be managed endoscopically.[61] These cases highlight the importance of objective anatomic evaluation in patients with new symptoms such as dysphagia.

One less morbid complication, which can still have a large impact on quality of life, is hyper flatulence. Bloating and hyper flatulence is relatively common after Nissen fundoplication. One study of 52 patients found that 39% of patients complained of hyper flatulence at 18 months after PEHR.[62] Fortunately, studies suggest that these symptoms tend to improve overtime.[63]

Complicated anatomy in conjunction with a technically difficult procedure puts patients at risk for iatrogenic cardiac injury, splenic complications, bleeding, and ischemia. One center reported a case of a male aged 80 years, who underwent emergent PEHR for gastric outlet obstruction, which was complicated by cardiovascular shock presenting on postoperative day 1 secondary to pericardial tamponade and was successfully treated with pericardiocentsis.[64] Another center reported a case of a patient who underwent PEHR complicated by pancreatic injury and leak, which ultimately required cystgastrostomy and

necrosectomy.[65] Other complications include case reports of ligation of the short gastric vessels leading to "wandering spleen", resulting in torsion and splenic infarction.[66]

SUMMARY

Paraesophageal hernia is a condition that disproportionately affects older patients and those with medical comorbidities. As a result, the patient population typically in need of PEHR is at a higher risk for general perioperative and postoperative complications (**Table 2**). However, PEHR is also a highly technical foregut procedure, requiring further consideration for the impact on foregut physiology. Acute perioperative reherniation may be rare, but because earlier reoperation is associated with better long-term symptomatic outcomes and fewer complications, data support early detection and repair, even if asymptomatic. By contrast, early and late reherniation is very common, but the majority do not cause symptoms and do not require reoperation. Leaks and perforations have far superior outcomes if detected and repaired intraoperatively. Postoperative detection frequently requires reoperation. However, some endoscopic interventions are available. Other complications such as gastroparesis or mesh-erosion may lead to multiple additional interventions. Comprehensive assessment of patient-specific risk is necessary for proper stratification and perioperative planning.

CLINICS CARE POINTS

- Acute perioperative reherniation after PEHR is often asymptomatic when identified on postoperative imaging. However, due to lower complication rates and superior outcomes, early repair of these acute recurrences is recommended.

- In contrast, management of delayed reherniation should include consideration for severity of presenting symptoms and type of hernia recurrence. Not all asymptomatic delayed recurrences require repair.

- Transient delayed gastric emptying is frequently seen in the early postoperative period following PEHR. Testing and treatment for gastroparesis should be reserved for patients with symptoms lasting longer than 2 to 3 months.

DISCLOSURE

The authors have nothing to disclose.

REFERENCES

1. Bowditch HI. A Treatise on Diaphragmatic Hernia: Being an Account of a Case Observed at the Massachusetts General Hospital; Followed by a Numerical Analysis of All the Cases of this Afection, Found Recorded in the Writings of Medical Authors, Between the Years 1610 and 1846. Jewett: Thomas; 1853.

2. Soresi AL. Diaphragmatic hernia: its unsuspected frequency: its diagnosis: technic for radical cure. Ann Surg 1919;69(3):254.

3. Skinner DB, Belsey RH, Russell PS. Surgical management of esophageal reflux and hiatus hernia: long-term results with 1,030 patients. J Thorac Cardiovasc Surg 1967;53(1):33–54.

4. Stylopoulos N, Gazelle GS, Rattner DW. Paraesophageal hernias: operation or observation? Ann Surg 2002;236(4):492.

5. Schlottmann F, Strassle PD, Patti MG. Surgery for benign esophageal disorders in the US: risk factors for complications and trends of morbidity. Surg Endosc 2018;32:3675–82.

6. DeMeester SR, Bernard L, Schoppmann SF, et al. Elective laparoscopic paraesophageal hernia repair leads to an increase in life expectancy over watchful waiting in asymptomatic patients: an updated markov analysis. Ann Surg 2024;279(2):267–75.

7. Lidor AO, Chang DC, Feinberg RL, et al. Morbidity and mortality associated with antireflux surgery with or without paraesophogeal hernia: a large ACS NSQIP analysis. Surg Endosc 2011;25:3101–8.

8. Mehta S, Boddy A, Rhodes M. Review of outcome after laparoscopic paraesophageal hiatal hernia repair. Surg Laparosc Endosc Percutaneous Tech 2006;16(5):301–6.

9. Luketich JD, Nason KS, Christie NA, et al. Outcomes after a decade of laparoscopic giant paraesophageal hernia repair. J Thorac Cardiovasc Surg 2010;139(2):395–404. e391.

10. Le Page P, Furtado R, Hayward M, et al. Durability of giant hiatus hernia repair in 455 patients over 20 years. Ann R Coll Surg Engl 2015;97(3):188–93.

11. Kamarajah SK, Boyle C, Navidi M, et al. Critical appraisal of the impact of surgical repair of type II–IV paraoesophageal hernia (POH) on pulmonary improvement: a systematic review and meta-analysis. Surgeon 2020;18(6):365–74.

12. Ballian N, Luketich JD, Levy RM, et al. A clinical prediction rule for perioperative mortality and major morbidity after laparoscopic giant paraesophageal hernia repair. J Thorac Cardiovasc Surg 2013;145(3):721–9.

13. Tam V, Luketich JD, Winger DG, et al. Non-elective paraesophageal hernia repair portends worse outcomes in comparable patients: a propensity-adjusted analysis. J Gastrointest Surg 2017;21:137–45.

14. Ferri L, Feldman L, Stanbridge D, et al. Should laparoscopic paraesophageal hernia repair be abandoned in favor of the open approach? Surgical Endoscopy And Other Interventional Techniques 2005;19:4–8.

15. Karmali S, McFadden S, Mitchell P, et al. Primary laparoscopic and open repair of paraesophageal hernias: a comparison of short-term outcomes. Dis Esophagus 2008;21(1):63–8.

16. Cocco A, Chai V, Read M, et al. Percentage of intrathoracic stomach predicts operative and postoperative morbidity, persistent reflux and PPI requirement following laparoscopic hiatus hernia repair and fundoplication. Surg Endosc 2023;37(3):1994–2002.

17. Liu DS, Wee MY, Grantham J, et al. Routine esophagograms following hiatus hernia repair minimizes reoperative morbidity: a multicenter comparative cohort study. Ann Surg 2022;276(6):e770. e77.

18. Tsunoda S, Jamieson GG, Devitt PG, et al. Early reoperation after laparoscopic fundoplication: the importance of routine postoperative contrast studies. World J Surg 2010;34:79–84.

19. Frantzides CT, Madan AK, Carlson MA, et al. A prospective, randomized trial of laparoscopic polyetrafluoroethylene (PTFE) patch repair vs simple cruroplasty for large hiatal hernia. Arch Surg 2002;137(6):649–52.

20. Oelschlager BK, Pellegrini CA, Hunter JG, et al. Biologic prosthesis to prevent recurrence after

laparoscopic paraesophageal hernia repair: long-term follow-up from a multicenter, prospective, randomized trial. J Am Coll Surg 2011;213(4):461–8.

21. Jobe BA, Aye RW, Deveney CW, et al. Laparoscopic management of giant type III hiatal hernia and short esophagus: objective follow-up at three years. J Gastrointest Surg 2002;6(2):181–8.

22. Zehetner J, DeMeester SR, Ayazi S, et al. Laparoscopic versus open repair of paraesophageal hernia: the second decade. J Am Coll Surg 2011; 212(5):813–20.

23. Hashemi M, Peters JH, DeMeester TR, et al. Laparoscopic repair of large type III hiatal hernia: objective followup reveals high recurrence rate. J Am Coll Surg 2000;190(5):553–60.

24. Schlottmann F, Strassle PD, Allaix ME, et al. Paraesophageal hernia repair in the USA: trends of utilization stratified by surgical volume and consequent impact on perioperative outcomes. J Gastrointest Surg 2017;21:1199–205.

25. Ayazi S, Chowdhury N, Zaidi AH, et al. Magnetic sphincter augmentation (MSA) in patients with hiatal hernia: clinical outcome and patterns of recurrence. Surg Endosc 2020;34:1835–46.

26. Buckley Fr, Bell RC, Freeman K, et al. Favorable results from a prospective evaluation of 200 patients with large hiatal hernias undergoing LINX magnetic sphincter augmentation. Surg Endosc 2018;32: 1762–8.

27. Sillcox R, Carrera R, Wright AS, et al. Esophageal motility patterns in paraesophageal hernia patients compared to sliding hiatal hernia: Bigger is not better. J Gastrointest Surg 2023;27(10):2039–44.

28. Saad AR, Velanovich V. Anatomic observation of recurrent hiatal hernia: recurrence or disease progression? J Am Coll Surg 2020;230(6):999–1007.

29. Mattar S, Bowers S, Galloway K, et al. Long-term outcome of laparoscopic repair of paraesophageal hernia. Surg Endosc 2002;16:745–9.

30. Furnée EJ, Draaisma WA, Simmermacher RK, et al. Long-term symptomatic outcome and radiologic assessment of laparoscopic hiatal hernia repair. Am J Surg 2010;199(5):695–701.

31. Schuchert MJ, Adusumilli PS, Cook CC, et al. The impact of scoliosis among patients with giant paraesophageal hernia. J Gastrointest Surg 2011;15: 23–8.

32. Schlosser KA, Maloney SR, Prasad T, et al. Mesh reinforcement of paraesophageal hernia repair: trends and outcomes from a national database. Surgery 2019;166(5):879–85.

33. Stadlhuber RJ, Sherif AE, Mittal SK, et al. Mesh complications after prosthetic reinforcement of hiatal closure: a 28-case series. Surg Endosc 2009;23: 1219–26.

34. Nandipati K, Bye M, Yamamoto SR, et al. Reoperative intervention in patients with mesh at the hiatus is associated with high incidence of esophageal resection—a single-center experience. J Gastrointest Surg 2013;17:2039–44.

35. Parker M, Bowers SP, Bray JM, et al. Hiatal mesh is associated with major resection at revisional operation. Surg Endosc 2010;24:3095–101.

36. Spiro C, Quarmby N, Gananadha S. Mesh-related complications in paraoesophageal repair: a systematic review. Surg Endosc 2020;34:4257–80.

37. Tog C, Liu D, Lim H, et al. Risk factors for delayed gastric emptying following laparoscopic repair of very large hiatus hernias. BJS open 2017;1(3): 75–83.

38. Strong AT, Landreneau JP, Cline M, et al. Per-oral pyloromyotomy (POP) for medically refractory postsurgical gastroparesis. J Gastrointest Surg 2019; 23:1095–103.

39. Lu D, Altieri MS, Yang J, et al. Investigating rates of reoperation or postsurgical gastroparesis following fundoplication or paraesophageal hernia repair in New York State. Surg Endosc 2019;33:2886–94.

40. Trus TL, Bax T, Richardson WS, et al. Complications of laparoscopic paraesophageal hernia repair. J Gastrointest Surg 1997;1(3):221–8.

41. Varvoglis DN, Farrell TM. Poor Gastric Emptying in Patients with Paraesophageal Hernias: Pyloroplasty, Per-Oral Pyloromyotomy, BoTox, or Wait and See? J Laparoendosc Adv Surg Tech 2022;32(11): 1134–43.

42. Hamrick MC, Davis SS, Chiruvella A, et al. Incidence of delayed gastric emptying associated with revisional laparoscopic paraesophageal hernia repair. J Gastrointest Surg 2013;17:213–7.

43. He S, Jia Y, Xu F, et al. Transient delayed gastric emptying following laparoscopic Nissen fundoplication for gastroesophageal reflux disease. Langenbeck's Arch Surg 2021;406:1397–405.

44. Zhang LP, Chang R, Matthews BD, et al. Incidence, mechanisms, and outcomes of esophageal and gastric perforation during laparoscopic foregut surgery: a retrospective review of 1,223 foregut cases. Surg Endosc 2014;28:85–90.

45. Urschel JD. Gastroesophageal leaks after antireflux operations. Ann Thorac Surg 1994;57(5):1229–32.

46. Mencio MA, Ontiveros E, Burdick JS, et al. Use of a novel technique to manage gastrointestinal leaks with endoluminal negative pressure: a single institution experience. Surg Endosc 2018;32:3349–56.

47. Murdock CM, Wolff AJ, Van Geem T. Risk factors for hypercarbia, subcutaneous emphysema, pneumothorax, and pneumomediastinum during laparoscopy. Obstet Gynecol 2000;95(5):704–9.

48. Falk GL, D'Netto TJ, Phillips S, et al. Pneumothorax: laparoscopic intraoperative management during fundoplication facilitates management of cardiopulmonary instability and surgical exposure. J Laparoendosc Adv Surg Tech 2018;28(11):1371–3.

49. Kaur R, Kohli S, Jain A, et al. Pneumothorax during laparoscopic repair of giant paraesophageal hernia. J Anaesthesiol Clin Pharmacol 2011;27(3):373.

50. Gogalniceanu P, Crewdson K, Khan A, et al. Transhiatal chest drainage after oesophagectomy. Ann R Coll Surg Engl 2007;89(5):535–6.

51. Ivy M, White P, Bograd A, et al. Topic: Esophagus Benign-GERD, Achalasia, Motility Abstract ID: 36 Pleurotomies During Minimally Invasive Anti-Reflux and Hiatal Hernia Repair are Not Associated With Higher Rates of Complications. Foregut 2023;3(3): 357–8.

52. Voyles CR, Madden B. The "floppy diaphragm" sign with laparoscopic-associated pneumothorax. J Soc Laparoendosc Surg: J Soc Laparoendosc Surg 1998;2(1):71.

53. Bujoreanu I, Abrar D, Lampridis S, et al. Do poor functional outcomes and higher morbidity following emergency repair of giant hiatus hernia warrant elective surgery in asymptomatic patients? Frontiers Surg 2021;8:628477.

54. Tang S-J, Tran T, Memmesheimer C, et al. Paraesophageal hernia repair and deep vein thrombosis. J Clin Gastroenterol 2002;34(2):187–8.

55. Klock JA, Walters RW, Nandipati KC. Robotic hiatal hernia repair associated with higher morbidity and readmission rates compared to laparoscopic repair: 10-year analysis from the National Readmissions Database (NRD). J Gastrointest Surg 2023;27(3): 489–97.

56. Ward MA, Hasan SS, Sanchez CE, et al. Complications following robotic hiatal hernia repair are higher compared to laparoscopy. J Gastrointest Surg 2021;1–7.

57. Gerull WD, Cho D, Kuo I, et al. Robotic approach to paraesophageal hernia repair results in low long-term recurrence rate and beneficial patient-centered outcomes. J Am Coll Surg 2020;231(5): 520–6.

58. O'Connor SC, Mallard M, Desai SS, et al. Robotic versus laparoscopic approach to hiatal hernia repair: results after 7 years of robotic experience. Los Angeles, CA: SAGE Publications Sage CA; 2020.

59. Soliman BG, Nguyen DT, Chan EY, et al. Robot-assisted hiatal hernia repair demonstrates favorable short-term outcomes compared to laparoscopic hiatal hernia repair. Surg Endosc 2020;34:2495–502.

60. Ma L, Luo H, Kou S, et al. Robotic versus laparoscopic surgery for hiatal hernia repair: a systematic literature review and meta-analysis. J Robot Surg 2023;1–12.

61. Rancourt M, Paré A, Comeau É. Case Report: Intraoesophageal migration of Teflon pledgets used for hiatal hernia repair: a serious adverse event. BMJ Case Rep 2019;12(4).

62. Swanstrom LL, Jobe BA, Kinzie LR, et al. Esophageal motility and outcomes following laparoscopic paraesophageal hernia repair and fundoplication. Am J Surg 1999;177(5):359–63.

63. Swanstrom L, Wayne R. Spectrum of gastrointestinal symptoms after laparoscopic fundoplication. Am J Surg 1994;167(5):538–41.

64. Cockbain AJ, Darmalingum A, Mehta SP. Acute deterioration after emergency paraesophageal hernia repair. Surgery 2016;159(6):1691–2.

65. Varda B, Jasurda J, Haseeb A. A rare case of paraesophageal hernia repair complicated by pancreatic injury. Cureus 2023;15(4).

66. Odabasi M, Abuoglu HH, Arslan C, et al. Asymptomatic partial splenic infarction in laparoscopic floppy Nissen fundoplication and brief literature review. Int Surg 2014;99(3):291–4.

Paraesophageal Hernias with Perforation

Adam H. Lackey, MD[a,b], Joanna Sesti, MD[b,*]

KEYWORDS

- Paraesophageal hernia complication • Gastric volvulus • Esophageal and gastric perforation
- Strangulated diaphragmatic hernia • Hiatal hernia

KEY POINTS

- Acute presentation of gastric volvulus is a rare condition which may be complicated by ischemia.
- Endoscopy is the mainstay for evaluating gastric mucosa for viability in patients with gastric volvulus.
- Computer-aided tomography can be useful in diagnosis of gastric volvulus with perforation.
- Tenets of surgical repair include reduction of the hernia, resection of devitalized tissue, and drainage.
- Damage control with esophageal exclusion may be necessary in case of hemodynamic instability.

INTRODUCTION AND PREVALENCE

Gastric volvulus is a rare condition characterized by the abnormal rotation of the stomach along its longitudinal (organoaxial) or transverse (mesenteroaxial) axis (**Fig. 1**). In the case of organoaxial volvulus, the proximal to distal orientation of the fundus and antrum are maintained, while in mesenteroaxial volvulus, this orientation can be distorted with the antrum or pylorus lying above the gastroesophageal (GE) junction.

Gastric volvulus can be seen in the setting of paraesophageal hernias. In 70% of cases, it can present with Borchardt's triad: severe epigastric pain, vomiting, and difficulty or inability to pass a nasogastric tube.[1–3] Strangulation is an uncommon complication occurring in less than one-third of cases and more often associated with the organoaxial subtype. Complications include ulceration, perforation, hemorrhage, pancreatic necrosis, and omental avulsion.[4–6] Mortality is as high as 42% to 56% without prompt intervention.[2,7]

DIAGNOSIS
Chest and Abdominal Radiography

Typical findings of gastric volvulus in chest radiograph include an intrathoracic, upside-down stomach as evidenced by mediastinal or retrocardiac air-fluid levels (**Fig. 2**). In the case of a complicated volvulus with perforation, pneumomediastium, pneumoperitoneum, or a pleural effusion may be appreciated. Upright abdominal radiographs can show an unexpected location of the gastric bubble, double air-filled level, a large, distended stomach, and/or collapsed small bowel.[8,9]

Fluoroscopy

Barium studies may show a distended stomach in the left upper quadrant extending into the thorax. The appearance of an inverted stomach will depend on the subtype of volvulus, that is, the antrum and pylorus may lie above the gastric fundus in case of mesenteroaxial volvulus. Luminal obstruction in case of >180° twists will show

[a] Thoracic Surgery, Robert Wood Johnson Barnabas Health, 101 Old Short Hills Road, Suite 302, West Orange, NJ 07052, USA; [b] Thoracic Surgery, Cooperman Barnabas Medical Center, Robert Wood Johnson Barnabas Health, Livingston, NJ, USA
* Corresponding author. 101 Old Short Hills Road, West Orange, NJ 07052.
E-mail address: Joanna.sesti@rwjbh.org

Thorac Surg Clin 34 (2024) 371–376
https://doi.org/10.1016/j.thorsurg.2024.06.003
1547-4127/24/© 2024 Elsevier Inc. All rights reserved, including those for text and data mining, AI training, and similar technologies.

A 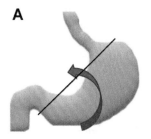   **B**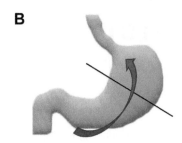

Fig. 1. Different types of gastric volvulus. (*A*) Organoaxial volvulus results from rotation along the long axis of the stomach from the gastroesophageal junction to the pylorus. (*B*) Mesenteroaxial volvulus results from rotation along the transverse axis such that the pylorus rotates above the gastroesophageal junction.

incomplete or absent entrance of contrast material into and/or out of the stomach (**Fig. 3**). A typical "beaking" may be demonstrated at the point of the twist.[8] Teague and colleagues suggested that barium studies are the most reliable in diagnosis of gastric volvulus with 14 out of 25 studies being diagnostic.[10]

Computer-Aided Tomography

Computer-aided tomography (CT) is expected to play a more important role in diagnosing gastric volvulus. Benefits of CT scan include 24-h access, speed, definition of the anatomic defect, assessment of gastric viability, and perforation.[4] Griffin and colleagues found CT to be more sensitive (100%) than endoscopy (84%) in diagnosis.[1] This is a relatively new development in the last 2 decades which challenges previous results as in the study by Teague and colleagues. CT findings of acute gastric volvulus were explored by Alili and colleagues[11] The most common findings in patients with surgically confirmed gastric volvulus included paraesophageal hernia (80%), AP transition point

with or without mass (100%), antrum at the same level or higher than the fundus (100%), and intrathoracic position of the antrum (90%) (**Fig. 4**). CT findings of ischemia and peroration can include perigastric fluid, pneumoperitoneum, pneumomediastinum, gastric wall pneumatosis, lack of gastric wall enhancement, and hepatic, splenic, or pancreatic ischemia (**Fig. 5**). No relationship between CT signs of ischemia and final bowel ischemia at pathology was seen by Alili and colleagues. Moreover, 5 patients with gastric wall pneumatosis had resolution of the latter after nasogastric aspiration on repeat CT.[11] Nevertheless, if signs of ischemia are noted on CT, imaging direct visualization via endoscopy or surgery should be considered.

Endoscopy

Upper endoscopy plays a diagnostic and potentially therapeutic role in the evaluation and management of gastric volvulus. Viability of the gastric wall can be assessed as well as areas of perforation. Although it is not always possible to

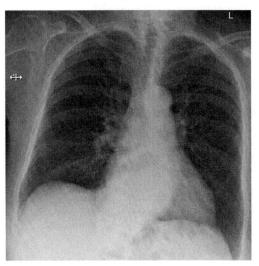

Fig. 2. Anterior-posterior (AP) x-ray of the chest demonstrating a large gastric volvulus with a mediastinal air fluid level.

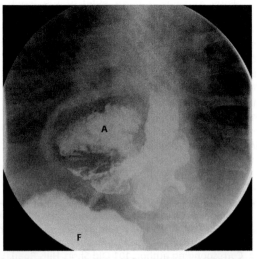

Fig. 3. Barium swallow of a patient with gastric volvulus and near complete obstruction. The stomach appears in 2 separate compartments separated by a small luminal tract. A, antrum; F, fundus.

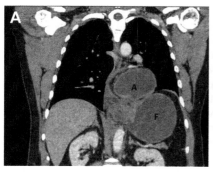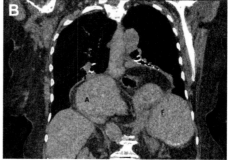

Fig. 4. (*A, B*) Computer-aided tomography of the chest in 2 patients with mesenteroaxial gastric volvulus. Note the inversion of the antrum and fundus in both images.

traverse the pylorus, some degree of decompression can be achieved.[1] If the stomach is viable and adequate decompression achieved with a nasogastric tube, semi-urgent intervention can be considered.

MANAGEMENT
Endoscopic Options

In general, endoscopy is more of a diagnostic tool for the complicated hiatal hernia than a therapeutic one. That being said, it is an integral part of the management of any hiatal hernia, including incarcerated, ischemic, and perforated hernias. In a patient who has some degree of incarceration or obstruction, or the rare patient with "mild" ischemia, there is a technique of endoscopic reduction of hernia that can be attempted, followed by percutaneous endoscopic gastrostomy (PEG) tube for fixation of the stomach in normal orientation.[12] However, this technique is something that few interventional gastrointestinal (GI)

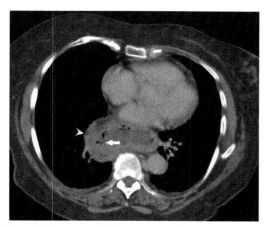

Fig. 5. Computer-aided tomography of the chest demonstrating gastric wall pneumatosis (*arrow*) and adjacent perigastric fluid with extraluminal air (*arrowhead*).

or surgery clinicians have familiarity with. Additionally, it is thought to have less success with increasing amounts of stomach herniated into the chest. The technique requires that the endoscope be navigated to the antrum and preferably post pyloric, and then suction is applied. The scope is then gently advance to push the fundus down into an intraabdominal position. Fluoroscopy can be helpful to assess the progress of moving the fundus into an intraabdominal position. Once the stomach is reduced, a PEG can be placed for fixation of the stomach in an intraabdominal, non-rotated configuration. If the stomach does not stay in an intraabdominal position as the scope is retracted, a second scope can be advanced inline for the purposes of PEG placement. This technique is obviously not appropriate for any patient with pre-existing perforation or frank ischemia and can clearly lead to perforation as a risk of the procedure.

As noted previously, in patients without a clear indication for emergent operative intervention such as perforation or necrosis, the first line of treatment is to decompress the distended stomach. Usual bedside "blind" placement of nasogastric tube (NGT) into the distended portion can be challenging due to the anatomy of the torsed stomach. Esophagogastroduodenoscopy (EGD) can be useful to help place the NGT in an optimal position, as long as no clear indication for surgery is noted at the time of endoscopy. There are several methods of accomplishing this, but this author's preference is to use an endoscopic snare. Briefly, the NGT is placed through the nares, and brought out through the mouth using direct laryngoscopy and a McGill forceps or Kelly clamp. A 0 silk suture is placed through the tip of the NGT, and it is usually helpful to have one end of the suture exiting the tip of the NGT. The suture is grasped with a snare or endoscopic forceps external to the patient's body, and then the EGD scope is reintroduced into the mouth and navigated to the desired location of the NGT. As the NGT presents an additional source of resistance to advancing the scope, it is sometimes helpful to independently feed the NGT into the nares as the scope is being advanced. Once the scope and NGT are at the desired location, the forceps is then released, or the snare can be briskly pulled on to break the suture.

Aside from the 2 techniques noted earlier, the role of endoscopy in an incarcerated hernia is mainly to diagnose if the patient has an indication for emergent surgical intervention. If the patient is noted to have perforation or frank ischemia, the endoscopy should be terminated at that point and the patient should be taken for surgical intervention. As most perforations occur as a result of distension and ischemia, efforts at advanced endoscopic techniques such as suturing and clipping will likely result in a closure of compromised tissue that would not be expected to be durable, at the expense of increased contamination from air insufflation and entrainment out of the perforation. Additionally, given that perforations may be venting into the peritoneum, mediastinum, or pleural space, the potential hemodynamic consequences of significant air insufflation into these spaces should be recognized, outside of the consequences of increased contamination that would occur during the prolonged air insufflation required for these advanced endoscopic techniques.

Although the argument for limited endoscopy is made earlier, it should be noted that once a patient has been noted to have a clear indication for surgical intervention, that is not the end of the role for endoscopy in these patients. Intraoperative EGD is essential during surgical intervention for several reasons. These include endoscopic evaluation of extent of ischemia once the stomach is reduced, evaluating any areas of resection or repair with an air leak test, and ensuring appropriate patency of the GI tract when proposed resection of compromised tissue is near the GE junction or in the antrum. Preoperative endoscopy can be omitted preoperatively in patients with a clear operative indication such as free air in the hernia sac or visible gastric wall discontinuity on CT, but should always be part of the overall operative management.

Surgical Management

Once a clear indication for emergent surgical intervention is identified, the patient should be expeditiously taken to the operating room. Resuscitation is frequently required for these patients, and should absolutely be undertaken, but should not significantly delay time to definitive intervention.

In all but the most moribund patients, surgical intervention is the mainstay of treatment. Larger hernias are more common in older, potentially more frail patients and more likely associated with complications such as incarceration and perforation. In the rare patient who is deemed truly too frail or ill for surgery, salvage with endoluminal vacuum dressing application or direct drainage has been described but should not be considered as standard of care.[13]

The surgical management of the ischemic or perforated stomach in the setting of hiatal hernia reflects the wide range of tissue compromise that can be found in these cases, ranging from reduction and second-look, direct debridement, and suture repair to wedge gastrectomy, total gastrectomy, and exclusion procedures.[14]

Surgical approach should be dictated by the clinical presentation and the comfort level of the operating surgeon. While hiatal hernias initially were repaired through a left thoracotomy, this has been supplanted in general by minimally invasive transabdominal approaches. Given some of the limitation of a transthoracic approach (inability to asses distal stomach and atrum, inability to perform gastropexy), a thoracotomy should be reserved for patients presenting with significant pleural or mediastinal contamination, in the hands of a surgeon with significant experience with hernia repair through the chest. Most repairs will be taken trans-abdominally, and the decision of laparoscopic vs open repair will depend as well on the operating surgeon's comfort level with advanced laparoscopic approaches. Patients presenting with gross and diffuse peritoneal contamination are probably best addressed with an open procedure. Outside of that scenario, a laparoscopic approach is reasonable as long as the surgeon is comfortable with laparoscopic foregut surgery and the patient will tolerate peritoneal insufflation, which is not necessarily a given since these patients can present dehydrated and in septic shock.

Regardless of the approach, the surgical principles are the same: reduction of the hernia, assessment of viability, resection of devitalized tissues, and repair of perforations. The assessment of devitalized tissue should be approached by both direct visualization as well as endoscopically. Overlay of any staple or suture lines with an omental flap is an easy and effective buttress of the repair. The appropriateness of formal repair of the hernia with resection of hernia sack and potentially fundoplication in the setting of ischemia or perforation is debatable, and should only be considered in the setting of hemodynamic stability and minimal soilage. In general, placement of mesh in the setting of a perforated stomach should be avoided, regardless if the mesh is biologic or permanent. It is very acceptable to resect any devitalized tissue, repair any perforations, perform a gastropexy or placement of G tube for fixation, and plan to return several months later for definitive repair of the hernia.

Any resection that occurs near the GE junction or the antrum should be undertaken with a bougie dilator or at least the EGD scope through the GE junction or pylorus, respectively, to ensure luminal patency. The surgeon should be aware that "second look" assessments of tissue viability are common in these situations, and very appropriate. Significant resection of the esophagus should be rare as this is generally an issue with gastric dilatation rather than a primary esophageal issue. In the relatively rare event that a patient requires a complete gastrectomy, there is usually enough viable esophagus that a esophago-jejunostomy can be entertained as a staged procedure. Given that surgical intervention in these situations usually involves intervention on ischemic or soiled foregut tissues in patients that are frequently frail or septic, consideration for a durable feeding access such as a jejunostomy tube should be considered, especially if the GI tract is in discontinuity at the time of initial intervention.

OUTCOMES

The most common complications following presentation with acute gastric volvulus include pneumonia and prolonged hospitalizations.[1] Analysis of individual records of the 1997 National Inpatient Sample (NIS) database showed only 27.6% of the patients undergoing emergency surgery had an uneventful recovery. Organ resection was necessary in 6.4% of the patients.[12] Published mortality rates of emergency surgery range from 5.4% to 40%. These rates are perhaps reflective of older techniques. More recent published reports show mortality rates around 1.1% versus 8% for elective versus emergency surgery. A 4-covariate (age >80, urgency or operation, congestive heart failure, and pulmonary disease) prediction model showed a discriminatory accuracy of 88% for mortality.[13,14]

SUMMARY

Hiatal hernia is a relatively common pathology that rarely requires urgent surgical intervention. In patients with acute obstruction, ischemia, or perforation, a low threshold for diagnostic procedures and therapeutic interventions may be able to salvage the patient. In patients with ischemia or perforation, standard surgical principles guide management and decision making. Once ischemia or perforation is identified, proceeding expeditiously to the operating room is usually the only intervention that can salvage the patient. In the setting of ischemia or perforation, formal repair of the hernia should be balanced with the patient's overall condition and the degree of soilage; the default choice should be deferring formal repair to a later date unless the patient is very stable and the soilage is minimal. The principles of second look for tissue at risk or staged procedures for patients in a compromised state are very appropriate in this unfortunate patient population. Elective repairs of large hernias are in general preferable to the risk of patients presenting in extremis—obstructed, ischemic, or perforated.

CLINICS CARE POINTS

- Gastric volvulus is characterized by the abnormal rotation of the stomch along its longitudinal or transverse axis.
- Computer aided tomography is an important diagnostic tool.
- Prompt diagnosis of ischemia and perforation followed by surgical intervention is paramount in improving rates of survival.

DISCLOSURE

The authors have no disclosures. This works was not supported by any funding or grants.

REFERENCES

1. Light D, Links D, Griffin M. The threatened stomach: management of the acute gastric volvulus. Surg Endosc 2016;30(5):1847–52.
2. Chau B, Dufel S. Gastric volvulus. Emerg Med J 2007;24(6):446–7.
3. Kur BM. Pathologie and Therapie des magen volvulus. Arch Kin Chir 1904;74:243–60.
4. Shivanand G, Seema S, Srivastava DN, et al. Gastric volvulus: acute and chronic presentation. Clin Imaging 2003;27(4):265–8.
5. Oh SK, Han BK, Levin TL, et al. Gastric volvulus in children: the twists and turns of an unusual entity. Pediatr Radiol 2008;38(3):297–304.

6. Estevao-Costa J, Soares-Oliveira M, Correia-Pinto J, et al. Acute gastric volvulus secondary to a Morgagni hernia. Pediatr Surg Int 2000;16(1–2):107–8.

7. Rashid F, Thangarajah T, Mulvey D, et al. A review article on gastric volvulus: a challenge to diagnosis and management. Int J Surg 2010;8(1):18–24.

8. Jones JE-FM, Chacko A. Gastric volvulus. 2009. Available at: https://radiopaedia.org/articles/6170.

9. Peterson CM, Anderson JS, Hara AK, et al. Volvulus of the gastrointestinal tract: appearances at multimodality imaging. Radiographics 2009;29(5):1281–93.

10. Teague WJ, Ackroyd R, Watson DI, et al. Changing patterns in the management of gastric volvulus over 14 years. Br J Surg 2000;87(3):358–61.

11. Millet I, Orliac C, Alili C, et al. Computed tomography findings of acute gastric volvulus. Eur Radiol 2014;24(12):3115–22.

12. Stylopoulos N, Gazelle GS, Rattner DW. Paraesophageal hernias: operation or observation? Ann Surg 2002;236(4):492–500. discussion 500-491.

13. Ballian N, Luketich JD, Levy RM, et al. A clinical prediction rule for perioperative mortality and major morbidity after laparoscopic giant paraesophageal hernia repair. J Thorac Cardiovasc Surg 2013;145(3):721–9.

14. Tam V, Luketich JD, Winger DG, et al. Non-Elective Paraesophageal Hernia Repair Portends Worse Outcomes in Comparable Patients: a Propensity-Adjusted Analysis. J Gastrointest Surg 2017;21(1):137–45.

Perforated Esophageal Cancer

Christopher Strader, MD, Shawn S. Groth, MD, MS*

KEYWORDS

- Esophageal carcinoma • Esophageal perforation • Treatment outcome

KEY POINTS

- A particularly challenging complication is perforated esophageal cancer, a surgical emergency that carries significant morbidity and mortality rates and dramatically changes the trajectory of a patient's cancer prognosis.
- The median survival from perforated esophageal cancer without esophagectomy is 2 months.
- In order to optimize the outcomes of such patients, early detection and prompt patient-centered management is essential. For highly select patients, esophagectomy is a reasonable treatment option.

INTRODUCTION

As the world's eighth most common cancer and its sixth most common cause of cancer-related death, esophageal carcinoma is both common and lethal. Consequently, health care providers who manage esophageal cancer patients, including thoracic surgeons, general surgeons, medical oncologists, radiation oncologists, gastroenterologists, intensivists, and emergency medicine physicians must possess a comprehensive understanding of the presentation, assessment, and management of complications of esophageal cancer treatment. A particularly challenging complication of esophageal cancer treatment is esophageal perforation, a surgical emergency that carries significant morbidity and mortality rates and dramatically changes the trajectory of a patient's cancer prognosis. In order to optimize the outcomes of such patients, early detection and prompt patient-centered management is essential.

Epidemiology

Worldwide, esophageal cancer ranks as the 8th highest in incident cancer cases and the 6th most common cause of cancer-related mortality, according to the World Health Organization-International Agency for Research on Cancer's data from Globocan 2020 to 2023.[1] In the United States (U.S.), there are over 21,000 new cases annually and over 16,000 deaths each year, making it the 11th most common cause of cancer-related mortality in the US.[1] Most patients are diagnosed with advanced disease.[2–4]

In general, esophageal perforation is rare (3.1 per 1,000,000). However, patients with esophageal cancer have a higher risk of perforation due to diagnostic endoscopy, palliative endoscopic interventions, and chemoradiation therapy.[5–7] Esophageal perforation complicates treatment in 5% to 8% of esophageal cancer patients undergoing palliative therapy.[6] The consequence is severe—25% to 50% of such perforations are fatal.[6–8] For those who survive, median survival is reduced to a mere 60 days, a nearly 90% reduction from the median 17 months survival with palliative radiation therapy in the absence of a perforation.[9]

ETIOLOGY

In general, esophageal perforation among esophageal cancer patients can be divided into 2 main

Division of Thoracic Surgery, Michael E. DeBakey Department of Surgery, Baylor College of Medicine, Houston, TX, USA
* Corresponding author. David J. Sugarbaker Division of Thoracic Surgery, Michael E. DeBakey Department of Surgery, 7200 Cambridge Street, Suite 6A, Houston, TX 77030.
E-mail address: Shawn.Groth@bcm.edu

Thorac Surg Clin 34 (2024) 377–383
https://doi.org/10.1016/j.thorsurg.2024.05.002
1547-4127/24/© 2024 Elsevier Inc. All rights are reserved, including those for text and data mining, AI training, and similar technologies.

groups based on their etiology: iatrogenic injury during diagnostic or palliative interventions and treatment-induced spontaneous perforation. Iatrogenic injury is much more common (60% of all such perforations) and carries a more favorable prognosis.[10–12] Treatment-induced spontaneous perforation is less common (1%–5% of perforations) and has a less favorable prognosis.[7,9,10]

Iatrogenic Perforation

From diagnosis and staging to palliation and symptom control, nearly every esophageal cancer patient will undergo one or more endoscopic procedures at some point during evaluation and treatment. The risk of iatrogenic perforation varies by the type of endoscope (ie, rigid vs flexible) being used and the endoscopic intervention being attempted.[7] Areas of the esophagus at the highest risk for perforation are those with luminal narrowing, whether they be anatomic (ie, Killian's triangle, the bronchoaortic constriction, or gastroesophageal junction) or pathologic (ie, malignant strictures).[10] **Table 1** lists several of the most common types of procedures and their associated risk of perforation. To the extent to which data is available in the literature, the reported values are based on the esophageal cancer patients. However, in many cases, there is a paucity of information when it comes to distinguishing between iatrogenic injury in benign or malignant disease.

The more favorable prognosis in the iatrogenic group is due to multiple factors, including patient age and comorbidities, early recognition during the procedure, and high vigilance in the immediate post-procedure period to recognize and intervene upon complications as early as possible in order to mitigate their impact.[13–24]

Treatment-Induced Spontaneous Perforation

Treatment-induced spontaneous perforation is a dreaded complication of chemoradiotherapy that carries a high mortality rate. Reported rates of spontaneous perforation during systemic therapy or chemoradiation therapy range from 5.6% to 28.1%.[9,18–21] Factors associated with an increased risk of spontaneous perforation include T4 tumors, esophageal stenosis, radiation therapy, re-irradiation, extracapsular lymph node invasion, age less than 60 to 65 years, squamous cell carcinoma, and ulcerative subtype.[9,18,20,22,23] Notably, for stage T1-T2 tumors, perforation from chemoradiotherapy is exceedingly rare but becomes more common with T3 and (particularly) T4 tumors.[23] One study found that the median interval from the time of intensity modulated radiotherapy to perforation was 4.4 months.[23] Prognosis after treatment-induced spontaneous perforation is poor - the median survival is only 2 months without surgery.[9]

CLINICAL PRESENTATION AND DIAGNOSIS

Esophageal perforation is a true surgical emergency, where mortality escalates as time elapses. In a recent systematic review, only 50% of patients will present within 24 hours of symptom onset, emphasizing the need for heightened vigilance among clinicians.[25] Patients with esophageal cancer are particularly susceptible to perforation due to factors such as endoscopic instrumentation, chemoradiotherapy, and advanced age.[9]

Clinical presentation of patients with esophageal perforation varies based on the location of the perforation and the amount of time that has elapsed since perforation occurred. Cervical esophageal perforations may manifest as neck pain, erythema, and edema, often associated with a recent history of endoscopic intervention. In contrast, perforations in the intrathoracic esophagus commonly present with chest pain, tachypnea, and shortness of breath. Perforations at the gastroesophageal junction are a particular diagnostic challenge, as they may exhibit intrathoracic symptomatology, intra-abdominal symptoms, or both. Notably, if evident on examination, subcutaneous emphysema may be a discernible sign of perforation.

With time, as the severity of the condition intensifies, signs and symptoms of sepsis or septic shock with multisystem organ failure may manifest.[26] A comprehensive history and physical examination are imperative, especially among esophageal cancer patients, as this will often yield clues to underlying etiology and location. In particular, when

Table 1
Common endoscopic interventions and their associated risk of perforation

Intervention	Risk of Perforation
Stent Without Radiotherapy[6,14]	6.1%
Stent With Radiotherapy[14]	9.4%
Endoscopic Mucosal Resection (EMR)[15]	0.3%–0.5%
Endoscopic Submucosal Dissection (ESD)[15,16]	4%–10%
Endoscopic Dilation[6,17]	1%–2%
Laser Therapy[6,8]	6%–10%
Radiofrequency Ablation (RFA)[24]	0.6%

obtaining the history of the esophageal cancer patient, details regarding stage at diagnosis, treatment timeline, and recent esophageal instrumentation are essential.

A full set of laboratory studies should be obtained, including a comprehensive metabolic panel, lactate, complete blood count, coagulation panel, and type and screen. A chest x-ray may reveal pertinent findings such as mediastinal air, pneumothorax or pleural effusion. In particular, the finding of pneumomediastinum should raise a high index of suspicion for an esophageal injury. However, the lack of pneumomediastinum does not rule out an esophageal injury, as its sensitivity has been reported to be as low as 26%.[27] For patients for whom an esophageal injury is on the differential, thoracic computed tomography (CT) with oral water-soluble contrast is useful. It has a high sensitivity and negative predictive value (both approaching 100%) and has the added value of assessing for mediastinal or pleural fluid collections that may require intervention. In the absence of a mediastinal or pleural fluid collection, pneumomediastinum or an overt esophageal wall defect, fluoroscopic esophagram can be omitted. However, if the index of suspicion for esophageal injury is high despite a lack of supportive findings on CT, a fluoroscopic esophagram with water soluble oral contrast should be obtained. If the fluoroscopic esophagram is negative with water-soluble contrast is normal, repeat fluoroscopic esophagram with thin barium will increase sensitivity such that a result negative for leak effectively rules out perforation. Of note, a water soluble contrast should be performed before a barium study, since barium is not water-soluble, and spillage into the chest or abdomen causes extreme local inflammation and adhesions and is exceedingly difficult to wash out after spillage occurs.

MANAGEMENT

Managing esophageal perforation in esophageal cancer patients presents a particular challenge for endoscopists and surgeons that requires balancing treatment goals with realistic prognostic expectations. After perforation, reported median survival rates are as short as 60 days.[9]

Further complicating management, mortality increases quickly as time elapses, which can limit the time available for shared decision-making discussions with patients and their loved ones on goals of care. This can lead to a limited understanding amongst patients and their families of the prognosis and long-term outcomes. Even without stratifying for malignancy, historical series have reported mortality rates for esophageal

perforations (benign and malignant) as high as 30% with treatment. However, more contemporary series suggest the mortality rate in the current era is 3% to 15%. To optimize the chance for survival from the immediate impact of perforated esophageal cancer, expeditious diagnosis and treatment are essential[25] Though the literature on mortality of esophageal perforation among esophageal cancer patients is limited, these rates are likely higher for cancer patients with underlying medical comorbidities that often include chronic malnutrition, functional decline, and immunosuppressive treatments.

It should be recognized that not all perforations are alike, varying from microperforations from endoscopic interventions in hemodynamically normal patients to large areas of devitalized tissue and undrained collections in immunosuppressed patients with septic shock and multisystem organ failure.

Initial Management

Management of all patients with esophageal perforation (benign or malignant) is the same–resuscitation according to oxygen transport criteria, source control, and metabolic support. One in four patients will develop sepsis, and initial stabilization and treatment should follow the Surviving Sepsis Campaign Guidelines, including aggressive goal-directed intravenous fluid resuscitation and empiric broad-spectrum IV antimicrobials, which includes coverage for aerobes, anaerobes, and fungus.[25] The next steps of treatment depend on the patient's goals of care, their clinical stability, the location and size of perforation, and the extent of contamination of the mediastinum and pleural spaces.

Non-operative Management

Observation and medical therapy alone
Reserved for stable patients with contained perforations with no extraluminal contamination, this strategy involves close monitoring and constant reevaluation over 48 hours, with immediate intervention if clinical status deteriorates. Patients should be made *nil per os* and started on empiric antimicrobial therapy. A change in clinical status or increased clinical concern warrants repeat imaging and immediate reevaluation.

Advanced endoscopy
Generally, there has been a shift over the past 2 decades toward increased utilization of advanced endoscopy as first-line treatment of esophageal perforation.[28] No randomized controlled trials exist comparing endoscopy and surgery. However, with

careful patient selection, endoscopic management has been demonstrated to be an effective alternative to surgery in the setting of benign disease. In contrast, the management of esophageal perforation of esophageal cancer patients is different from those with benign perforations, and the utility of endoscopic interventions is much more limited. Perforations through neoplastic tissue cannot undergo the processes necessary to heal properly, and most advanced endoscopic techniques (eg, endoscopic clipping or suturing) are contraindicated.[22] Fully covered esophageal stent placement or endoluminal vacuum therapy are both palliative options to minimize sepsis but are unlikely to promote fistula resolution.

"Nonoperative" hybrid treatment It is well-established that esophageal stenting is safe, easy to use, and an effective alternative to surgical treatment in select cases of esophageal perforation.[28] In addition to being less invasive than surgical intervention, stenting has an advantage of allowing patients to get back to taking oral nutrition earlier.[29] Stents are typically left in place for 2 to 4 weeks, after which the stent is removed, the area re-evaluated, and the stent replaced until the excluded area has healed.

In contrast to patients with benign perforations or leaks after esophagectomy, the use of stents for perforated esophageal cancer is limited by several factors. First, because the tissues surrounding the perforation are neoplastic, healing is impaired, leading to longer times for the perforation to heal (if at all), translating into longer stent-dwelling times and increased stent-related complications. Second, for patients undergoing systemic therapy and/or radiation therapy, multidisciplinary discussions with medical and radiation oncology are necessary to determine whether further therapy can be given, balancing the need to deliver cancer-directed therapy with the risks of complications in an immunosuppressed cancer patient from an esophageal fistula that is unlikely to heal without resection. As such, we recommend that esophageal stenting only be employed in patients whose goals are palliative and when systemic therapy is no longer an option or part of their desired treatment plan. In such cases, endoscopic stenting is a viable alternative to aggressive surgical intervention by limiting sepsis and allowing early resumption of P.O. intake without the pain and time to recover from surgery.

A variety of fully covered stents is available and can be placed over a guidewire under endoscopic or fluoroscopic visualization or can be placed through the working channel of a therapeutic scope. A key concept for stent success is adequate proximal and distal mucosal apposition to the stent, in order to the effectively exclude the defect. In general, stent effectiveness is reduced as the size of the perforation increases (>6 cm) and are more challenge to use near the upper esophageal sphincter and gastroesophageal junction. If the perforation involves the proximal cervical esophagus, a stent may be poorly tolerated, as they can evoke a gagging sensation. At the gastroesophageal junction, the diameter of the proximal stomach flares and given the wider diameter of the proximal stomach, the stent becomes unable to align with the 2 different diameters. As such, esophageal stents are most effective in the tubular esophagus; perforations of the cervical esophagus and gastroesophageal junction typically require alternative management strategies. Stents may be used alone or in conjunction with drainage of mediastinal or pleural fluid collections. Because fully covered stents may migrate, we suggest fixing them in place with endoscopic sutures or through-the-scope clips and monitoring for migration with serial chest x-rays.

Operative Management

Patients with full-thickness esophageal perforation through neoplastic tissue should be classified as having carcinomatosis, which should factor into goals of care discussions[30] In contrast to those patients with benign esophageal perforations where primary repair is the gold standard, patients with perforated esophageal cancer typically require esophagectomy. For patients with perforations who are deemed to be appropriate candidates for aggressive surgical intervention, we typically recommend a 2-stage procedure with esophagectomy and diversion (first stage), followed by delayed reconstruction after adjuvant therapy (second stage), as cancer patients are at a higher risk of complications and any complications will delay recovery and the resumption of systemic and/or radiation therapy.

2-stage procedure

For most patients, a 2-stage procedure is safest, allowing them time to recover and return to their baseline status prior to performing the reconstruction. Delaying reconstruction also permits earlier initiation of adjuvant therapy and avoids delays of care due to anastomotic complications. Hard indications for the 2-stage approach include hemodynamic instability, sepsis, locally advanced disease (eg, spontaneously perforated at tumor site), significant contamination, or malnutrition.

Generally, we choose to enter the chest on the side of the perforation to allow simultaneous drainage/decortication of mediastinal or pleural collections while mobilizing the esophagus from the thoracic inlet to the hiatus. We then enter the abdomen, and staple off the proximal stomach, distal to the tumor. The hiatus is closed to prevent hiatal herniation. A venting gastrostomy tube is placed near the lesser curvature to avoid compromising the construction of the gastric conduit during esophageal reconstruction. A feeding jejunostomy tube is placed. Depending on the surgeon's experience and the degree of patient stability, the operation's thoracic and abdominal phase can be performed in a minimally invasive fashion. Finally, a cervical esophagostomy is constructed. Depending on the patient's stability, bipolar esophageal exclusion can be performed in a staged fashion.

Single-stage procedure
In highly select cases, a single-stage esophagectomy and immediate reconstruction may be considered, especially those patients with early-stage disease, with minimal contamination, and who are hemodynamically normal. Such cases are typically limited to otherwise fit individuals undergoing workup for an esophageal mass and suffer an iatrogenic injury during workup or attempted endoscopic resection. For those with sepsis or significant contamination, a 2-stage approach is safer.

In these highly select cases for which a single-stage procedure is chosen, the approach (transthoracic or transhiatal) and technique (minimally invasive, open, or hybrid), route (posterior mediastinal vs substernal) depends on the degree of pleural contamination (if present a transthoracic open is preferred) and surgeon experience and preference. If immediate reconstruction is performed in a patient with perforated esophageal cancer, a tubularized gastric conduit should be used for esophageal reconstruction, as colon graft (which require bowel preparation) and jejunal free grafts (which require microvascular anastomoses) have added complexity that are best suited for purely elective reconstructions. It is prudent to construct the anastomosis outside the area of contamination, which typically necessitates a cervical anastomosis. Consequently, for perforated distal esophageal/gastroesophageal junction carcinomas roux-en-Y reconstructions are also generally ill-advised.

Minimally invasive versus open esophagectomy
The safety, feasibility, and advantages of elective minimally invasive esophagectomy have been well-documented.[31] Indeed, level I evidence from 3 randomized controlled trials, multiple meta-analyses and an abundance of observational data indicate that elective minimally invasive esophagectomy for (nonperforated) esophageal cancer is associated with less complications than open approaches without compromising the oncologic quality and has durable quality-of-life benefits. However, the current literature regarding the use of minimally invasive approaches specifically for cases of perforations is limited to case reports and small case series.[32–34] As such, the current level of evidence suggests that the surgical approach should be based on the surgeon experience and the patient's clinical status, as hemodynamic instability and inability to tolerate single lung ventilation are contraindications to minimally invasive approaches.

Outcomes
There is a paucity of information in the contemporary literature on the outcomes following surgical resection for esophageal perforation in esophageal cancer patients. A single institution study from Canada, noted a striking 30-day mortality rate of 63% for such patients.[35] Indeed, the odds of 30-day mortality were 20-fold higher for patients with malignant perforations, a somber reminder of the severity of esophageal perforations in patients with carcinoma, likely due to the patients underlying clinical status, including the degree of immunosuppression and malnutrition. For patients with perforated esophageal cancer treated conservatively with an esophageal stent, the median survival is also poor–2 months.[9] Nonetheless, esophagectomy remains a reasonable option to manage malignant esophageal perforations in highly select patients who were potential candidates for esophagectomy prior to the perforation, especially those patients who had a reasonable chance of survival prior to the perforation (eg, patients who responded to chemoradiation therapy) given recent advances in systemic therapy for advanced disease.[36]

SUMMARY

The overall prognosis for patients with esophageal malignancy remains poor. The majority of patients with esophageal cancer present with advanced disease and are not surgical candidates at the time of diagnosis. Currently, for patients who present with malignant esophageal perforation, multiple treatment pathways exist spanning the spectrum from strictly non-interventional end-of-life care, to hybrid palliation with stent and drainage to surgical resection and adjuvant therapy in highly select patients. The treatment choice must be weighed against the poor prognosis among such patients. Given the complexity of factors that must be weighed, choosing which pathway to pursue should center around a shared decision model between experienced clinicians and patients and their families.

CLINICS CARE POINTS

- There is a lack of strong evidence in the literature to guide treatment of perforated esophageal cancer.
- Consequently, evidence-based treatment is extrapolated from the treatment of benign perforations in the context of prognosis for such patients.
- Esophageal stenting for a malignant perforation is palliative and is unlikely to heal.
- Esophagectomy is a reasonable treatment approach for highly selected patients and should typically done with bipolar exclusion and delayed reconstruction.

DISCLOSURE

Dr Shawn Groth discloses that he is a proctor for Intuitive Surgical Inc., Sunnyvale, CA.

REFERENCES

1. World Health Organization-International Agency for Research on Cancer. Global cancer data - Globocan 2020," 4 October 2023. Online. Available at: https://www.uicc.org/news/global-cancer-data-globocan-2018#:~:text=GLOBOCAN%202018%20is%20an%20online,for%20all%20cancer%20sites%20combined.
2. Enzinger PC, Mayer RJ. Esophageal cancer. N Engl J Med 2003;349(23):2241–52.
3. Rubenstein JH, Shaheen NJ. Epidemiology, Diagnosis, and Management of Esophageal Adenocarcinoma. Gastroenterology 2015;149(2):302–17.e1.
4. Kamarajah SK, Navidi M, Wahed S, et al. Significance of Neoadjuvant Downstaging in Carcinoma of Esophagus and Gastroesophageal Junction. Ann Surg Oncol 2020;27(9):3182–92.
5. Vidarsdottir H, Blondal S, Alfredsson H, et al. Oesophageal perforations in Iceland: a whole population study on incidence, aetiology and surgical outcome. Thorac Cardiovasc Surg 2010;58(8):476–80.
6. Morgan RA, Ellul JP, Denton ER, et al. Malignant esophageal fistulas and perforations: management with plastic-covered metallic endoprostheses. Radiology 1997;204(2):527–32.
7. Ferguson MK. Esophageal perforation and caustic injury: management of perforated esophageal cancer. Dis Esophagus 1997;10(2):90–4.
8. Tyrrell MR, Trotter GA, Adam A, et al. Incidence and management of laser-associated oesophageal perforation. Br J Surg 1995;82(9):1257–8.
9. Chen HY, Ma XM, Ye M, et al. Esophageal perforation during or after conformal radiotherapy for esophageal carcinoma. J Radiat Res 2014;55(5):940–7.
10. Brinster CJ, Singhal S, Lee L, et al. Evolving options in the management of esophageal perforation. Ann Thorac Surg 2004;77(4):1475–83.
11. Jones WG 2nd, Ginsberg RJ. Esophageal perforation: a continuing challenge. Ann Thorac Surg 1992;53(3):534–43.
12. Skinner DB, Little AG, DeMeester TR. Management of esophageal perforation. Am J Surg 1980;139(6):760–4.
13. Montminy EM, Jones B, Heller JC, et al. Endoscopic iatrogenic esophageal perforation and management: a retrospective outcome analysis in the modern era. BMC Gastroenterol 2023;23(1):371.
14. Tinusz B, Soós A, Hegyi P, et al. Efficacy and safety of stenting and additional oncological treatment versus stenting alone in unresectable esophageal cancer: A meta-analysis and systematic review. Radiother Oncol 2020;147:169–77.
15. ASGE technology committee, Kantsevoy SV, Adler DG, et al. Endoscopic mucosal resection and endoscopic submucosal dissection. Gastrointest Endosc 2008;68(1):11–8.
16. Noguchi M, Yano T, Kato T, et al. Risk factors for intraoperative perforation during endoscopic submucosal dissection of superficial esophageal squamous cell carcinoma. World J Gastroenterol 2017;23(3):478–85.
17. Takahashi H, Arimura Y, Okahara S, et al. Risk of perforation during dilation for esophageal strictures after endoscopic resection in patients with early squamous cell carcinoma. Endoscopy 2011;43(3):184–9.
18. Ohtsu A, Boku N, Muro K, et al. Definitive chemoradiotherapy for T4 and/or M1 lymph node squamous cell carcinoma of the esophagus. J Clin Oncol 1999;17(9):2915–21.
19. Kawakami T, Tsushima T, Omae K, et al. Risk factors for esophageal fistula in thoracic esophageal squamous cell carcinoma invading adjacent organs treated with definitive chemoradiotherapy: a monocentric case-control study. BMC Cancer 2018;18(1):573.
20. Kaneko K, Ito H, Konishi K, et al. Definitive chemoradiotherapy for patients with malignant stricture due to T3 or T4 squamous cell carcinoma of the oesophagus. Br J Cancer 2003;88(1):18–24.
21. Miyata H, Yamasaki M, Kurokawa Y, et al. Clinical relevance of induction triplet chemotherapy for esophageal cancer invading adjacent organs. J Surg Oncol 2012;106(4):441–7.
22. Zhu C, Wang S, You Y, et al. Risk Factors for Esophageal Fistula in Esophageal Cancer Patients Treated

with Radiotherapy: A Systematic Review and Meta-Analysis. Oncol Res Treat 2020;43(1–2):34–41.

23. Pao TH, Chen YY, Chang WL, et al. Esophageal fistula after definitive concurrent chemotherapy and intensity modulated radiotherapy for esophageal squamous cell carcinoma. PLoS One 2021;16(5): e0251811.

24. Qumseya BJ, Wani S, Desai M, et al. Adverse Events After Radiofrequency Ablation in Patients With Barrett's Esophagus: A Systematic Review and Meta-analysis. Clin Gastroenterol Hepatol 2016;14(8):1086–95.e6.

25. Sdralis EIK, Petousis S, Rashid F, et al. Epidemiology, diagnosis, and management of esophageal perforations: systematic review. Dis Esophagus 2017;30(8):1–6.

26. Khaitan PG, Famiglietti A, Watson TJ. The Etiology, Diagnosis, and Management of Esophageal Perforation. J Gastrointest Surg 2022;26(12):2606–15.

27. Caceres M, Cole FH, Weiman D. Clinical Pearls in Nonpenetrating Pneumomediastinum. Chest 2006; 130(4):270S.

28. Gurwara S, Clayton S. Esophageal Perforations: An Endoscopic Approach to Management. Curr Gastroenterol Rep 2019;21(11):57.

29. Homs MY, Steyerberg EW, Eijkenboom WM, et al. Single-dose brachytherapy versus metal stent placement for the palliation of dysphagia from oesophageal cancer: multicentre randomised trial. Lancet 2004;364(9444):1497–504.

30. Watkins AA, Zerillo JA, Kent MS. Trimodality Approach for Esophageal Malignancies. Surg Clin North Am 2021;101(3):453–65.

31. Ruurda JP, van der Sluis PC, van der Horst S, et al. Robot-assisted minimally invasive esophagectomy for esophageal cancer: A systematic review. J Surg Oncol 2015;112(3):257–65.

32. Nguyen NT, Follette DM, Roberts PF, et al. Thoracoscopic management of postoperative esophageal leak. J Thorac Cardiovasc Surg 2001;121(2):391–2.

33. Scott HJ, Rosin RD. Thoracoscopic repair of a transmural rupture of the oesophagus (Boerhaave's syndrome). J R Soc Med 1995;88(7):414P–5P.

34. Pickering O, Pucher PH, De'Ath H, et al. Minimally Invasive Approach in Boerhaave's Syndrome: Case Series and Systematic Review. J Laparoendosc Adv Surg Tech 2021;31(11):1254–61.

35. Bhatia P, Fortin D, Inculet RI, et al. Current concepts in the management of esophageal perforations: a twenty-seven year Canadian experience. Ann Thorac Surg 2011;92(1):209–15.

36. Soror T, Kho G, Zhao KL, et al. Impact of pathological complete response following neoadjuvant chemoradiotherapy in esophageal cancer. J Thorac Dis 2018;10(7):4069–76.

Aorto-esophageal Fistula Management

Leah J. Schoel, MD*, Kiran Lagisetty, MD

KEYWORDS

- Aorto-esophageal fistula • Aortic complications • Esophageal complications

KEY POINTS

- Aorto-esophageal fistulas (AEFs) are rare cardiovascular etiologies of upper gastrointestinal bleeding.
- AEFs are highly lethal and require prompt recognition and diagnosis.
- Thoracic endovascular aortic repair (TEVAR) may be used for initial hemorrhage control and bridging to definitive repair.
- The use of TEVAR alone is associated with high mid-term and long-term mortality and should not be considered definitive surgery for AEF.
- Open surgery with aortic graft replacement and esophagectomy has the highest reported 1 year survival rates.

INTRODUCTION

Aorto-esophageal fistula (AEF), a direct communication between the aorta and esophagus, is a rare and highly fatal condition, in which high-pressure aortic blood hemorrhages into the esophagus.[1] AEFs are a rare cardiovascular etiology of massive upper gastrointestinal bleeding (UGIB), comprising less than 1% of all massive UGIB, and AEFs comprise approximately 10% of these AEFs.[2] The annual incidence of AEF is approximately 1.5 per million.[3,4]

The first identified case of AEF was described in 1818 by a French naval surgeon named Dubrueil,[5] and the first survival of AEF reported was in 1980.[6] Prior to this survival, all 86 previously reported cases of AEF, which were secondary to foreign body in the esophagus, had been fatal.[7] When describing AEF from foreign body ingestion, Chiari defined the now classic Chiari's triad: (1) mid-thoracic pain or dysphagia, (2) sentinel episode of hematemesis, and (3) symptom-free interval followed by subsequent massive hematemesis with risks of exsanguination.[8,9] In this article, the authors review the major considerations, etiologies, diagnostics, and management of AEF, as well as ongoing controversies and future directions.

CONSIDERATIONS
Mortality

The morbidity and mortality following AEF are extremely high. Without operative intervention, AEF is universally fatal.[3,10] Even with intervention, in-hospital mortality rates have been reported up to 42%, and open operative mortality rates have been reported to reach 40%.[10–14] Given the lethality and severity of this condition, the need for rapid diagnosis and early intervention cannot be under-emphasized. A discussion with the patient and associated family or decision-makers regarding the prognosis and projected extent of care should be held immediately. Coordinated multidisciplinary care and communication is paramount.

Etiologies

AEF can be broadly categorized into primary and secondary. A primary AEF develops in a native

Department of Surgery, University of Michigan, Ann Arbor, MI, USA
* Corresponding author. Department of Surgery, University of Michigan, 1500 East Medical Center Drive, Ann Arbor, MI 48109.
E-mail address: leschoel@med.umich.edu

Thorac Surg Clin 34 (2024) 385–394
https://doi.org/10.1016/j.thorsurg.2024.07.004
1547-4127/24/© 2024 Elsevier Inc. All rights are reserved, including those for text and data mining, AI training, and similar technologies.

aorta, usually due to an aortic aneurysm, and less frequently due to foreign bodies and esophageal cancer, whereas a secondary AEF develops after the placement of endovascular prostheses, stent-grafts into the aorta, or placement of esophageal stents.[15,16] **Box 1** summarizes potential underlying causes of AEF.

In 1991, Hollander and Quick reviewed 500 AEF cases, and at that time, thoracic aortic aneurysms were found to be the most common etiology, representing 54% of cases.[3] Since this review, the most common etiology of AEF has changed, with prior intervention for aortic disease being most common.[14] This is now followed by thoracic aortic aneurysm, foreign body ingestion, thoracic malignancies (especially esophageal), and esophageal procedures (eg, esophageal stenting).[14] Other infrequent causes include trauma, infection (such as tuberculosis), or congenital anomalies of the great vessels.[14]

These changing etiologies are theorized to be secondary to increasing endovascular aortic interventions, esophageal procedures, and subsequent iatrogenic complications.[14] Endovascular aortic procedures that can precipitate AEF include thoracic endovascular aortic repair (TEVAR) or graft replacement, and esophageal procedures that can precipitate AEF include esophageal stenting.

> **Box 1**
> **Etiologies of aorto-esophageal fistula**
>
> Postoperative status for aortic disease
>
>   TEVAR
>
>   Thoracic aneurysm graft/repair
>
> Aortic aneurysm
>
> Foreign body ingestion
>
>   Bones—chicken, fish, steak
>
>   Razor blades/sharp objects
>
> Thoracic cancer
>
>   Esophageal carcinoma
>
> Postoperative status for esophageal disease
>
>   Esophageal stent
>
> Trauma
>
> Infectious
>
>   Mediastinal tuberculosis
>
>   History of syphilis
>
>   Esophagitis
>
> Congenital cardiac anomalies
>
> Caustic ingestion

The mean age of patients who develop AEF varies by etiology. The mean age is reported as 65.1 years for postoperative status for aortic disease, 67.2 years for aortic aneurysm, 60.4 years for thoracic cancer, and 47.9 years for foreign body ingestion.[14] As demonstrated here, the mean age of patients with AEF secondary to foreign body ingestion is significantly younger than that of patients with AEF from other causes.

Thoracic Endovascular Aortic Repair

The exact mechanisms of AEF formation complicating TEVAR are unknown. Stent-graft infection is considered to be a prominent mechanism of fistula formation.[17,18] Other hypotheses include (1) direct erosion of the relatively rigid stent-graft through the aorta into the esophagus; (2) pressure necrosis of the esophageal wall due to the continuing forces of the self-expanding endoprosthesis; (3) ischemic esophageal necrosis due to stent-graft coverage of aortic side branches that feed the esophagus; and (4) esophageal pressure from over-sizing the stent-graft device or an enlarging residual aneurysm.[17–21]

In another retrospective study, AEF formation following TEVAR was seen in patients who had developed mediastinal hematoma at the time of TEVAR,[18] which the authors hypothesized contributes to AEF formation through secondary esophageal ischemia and inflammation. To attenuate this devastating complication, these surgeons implemented a practice change with an elective left-sided mini-thoracotomy on the second day after TEVAR with a broad opening of the mediastinal pleura in order to decompress the posterior mediastinum.[18]

The timing between TEVAR and subsequent AEF formation ranges widely. In a large review, the median time between TEVAR and AEF presentation was 22.4 months[14]; however, in another large study, the median time interval was 90 days.[18]

Foreign Body Ingestion

AEF is a rare and highly dangerous complication of foreign body ingestion. Foreign bodies tend to be lodged at the level of the aortic arch, where the aortic arch presses against the esophagus and creates a relatively narrow lumen.[22,23] The mechanism of AEF formation after foreign body ingestion involves the gradual corrosion and subsequent piercing of the aortic wall by the foreign body. This is followed by pseudoaneurysm formation, extensive necrosis, and secondary infection.[24] Nandi and colleagues[7] followed up 2394 cases of impacted esophageal foreign bodies, and 2 (0.08%) cases developed an AEF. Lai and colleagues[25] looked at a consecutive series of 1338 foreign body ingestion, and none developed an AEF. Thus, while AEF is an extremely rare complication of foreign body ingestion, foreign bodies remain a leading cause of AEF.

The diagnosis and management of AEF after foreign body ingestion can be challenging. The history of foreign body ingestion may not always be available, and some patients may not recall ingesting the foreign body (ie, fish bones). Additionally, the interval between ingestion and clinical symptoms varies, ranging from days to more than 1 week,[23] and the symptomatology may be vague and may not correlate with the aortic or esophageal damage.[23]

OBSERVATION/ASSESSMENT/EVALUATION
Signs and Symptoms of Aorto-esophageal Fistula

The presentation of an AEF may vary widely, contributing to challenges in prompt diagnosis. Approximately 45% of patients present with all 3 components of Chiari's triad.[3,24,26,27] Midthoracic pain is reported in 59% of patients; sentinel hemorrhage is identified in 65% of patients; and the symptom-free interval has been described in up to 80% of patients.[3,27] The symptom-free interval may be due to arterial wall spasm, periaortic hematoma, or intravascular hypotension.[3]

In addition to the classic Chiari's triad, major clinical signs and symptoms at presentation include bright red hematemesis, dysphagia, backache, melena, fever, and shock,[26,28] which are common among all patients experiencing massive UGIB. Per reports, dysphagia is present in 45% of patients with AEF.[27] In some patients, fatal hemorrhage may be the presenting clinical symptom.[29] Tachycardia may not be present in patients taking a beta-blocker or calcium channel blocker. **Table 1** gives a summary of signs and symptoms of AEF. Given this wide spectrum of presentation, maintaining a high threshold of suspicion for an aortoenteric fistula is paramount. The interval between sentinel hemorrhage and fatal exsanguination can extend beyond 24 hours, and this "window of opportunity" should prompt rapid transfer of the patient to a center with advanced capabilities for managing the AEF.

It is important to ask patients suspected of AEF about previous endovascular or esophageal procedures, cancer, radiation to the neck, known aneurysmal disease, aspiration/ingestion, and other associated risk factors. Depending on the patient's presentation and chief complaints, the differential diagnosis is often broad and includes common causes of UGIB (eg, peptic ulcer disease and esophageal varices) and cardiac etiologies

Table 1
Signs and symptoms of aorto-esophageal fistula

Chiari's Triad	Midthoracic pain Sentinel hemorrhage Symptom-free interval followed by massive hemorrhage
Bright Red Hematemesis	May be massive, pulsatile, from mouth and nares
Pain	Back pain Anterior chest pain radiating to neck Retrosternal pain
Systemic Symptoms	Fever Tachycardia Malaise Fatigue may progress to lethargy
Gastrointestinal Symptoms	Dysphagia
Shock	Hemorrhagic Septic

(eg, acute myocardial infarction and aortic dissection). The diagnosis may not be obvious, and the symptomatology may be confusing; however, suspicion for AEF must remain high in patients with reports of hematemesis and concurrent gastrointestinal (GI) symptoms.

Principles of Management

Across the spectrum of clinical presentation, initial management of suspected AEF should consist of resuscitation and stabilization, per any UGIB.[2] There should be immediate establishment of 2 reliable large-bore intravenous (IVs; 14–18 gauge), fluid and blood product resuscitation, central venous access, arterial line placement, and intensive medical support. Laboratories including complete blood count (CBC), basic metabolic panel (BMP), blood cultures, arterial blood gas, type and crossmatch, and a coagulation panel should be sent immediately.

In the setting of massive hematemesis, securing a definitive airway is a critical priority.[2] However, patients with massive GIB are at risk of peri-intubation cardiovascular collapse, and resuscitation should take place before intubation, as able. The need for obtaining a secure airway will be dictated by the patient's clinical status.

Early blood product administration is a cornerstone of the management of massive UGIB, and prompt recognition and correction of any coagulopathy should follow. Although restrictive transfusion strategies target hemoglobin of 7 g/dL with an acute UGIB, massive GI hemorrhage requires aggressive resuscitation with prompt transfusion of blood products.[2,30] It is important to recognize that blood loss may not be accurately reflected in a CBC, as hemoglobin/hematocrit measurements lag behind the true serum concentration and are not reliable during acute massive GIB. A massive transfusion protocol with balanced transfusion should be initiated if the patient's clinical instability does not improve.[2,30]

Blood transfusion should be prioritized over crystalloid, as excessive crystalloid resuscitation may worsen anemia, contribute to developing coagulopathy, and increase acidosis.[31,32] Massive transfusion may precipitate hypocalcemia and hyperkalemia. Consider empiric calcium administration and monitor calcium levels throughout resuscitation. Similarly, potassium levels should be monitored, and hyperkalemia should be treated as indicated.

Thromboelastography (TEG) or rotational thromboelastometry (ROTEM) should be used to guide transfusion of blood products tailored to the patient's specific coagulopathy needs.[2,33] TEG and ROTEM provide vital dynamic information on coagulation, clot strength, and fibrinolysis; alterations in these laboratories signal the need for specific products such as platelets, cryoprecipitate, or fresh frozen plasma.[33]

Infection control with broad-spectrum antibiotics and antifungals should be administered, especially for patients with a prior history of endovascular stent placement. The specific combination may vary by institution and resistance patterns, but common combinations include meropenem, vancomycin, and fluconazole.[14] A collaboration with infectious disease experts and culture results should guide medical therapy. Lastly, considerations regarding nutritional needs will vary by both choice and timing of operative intervention; however, early consideration of nutrition is advisable. **Table 2** provides a summary of management needs for treatment of AEF.

Diagnostic Evaluation

On initial evaluation, history and physical will be performed as the patient's condition allows. Diagnostic workup will consist of laboratories and imaging. Laboratories including CBC, serum chemistry, 2 sets of blood cultures, arterial and/or venous blood gas, coagulation panel, type and crossmatch, and ROTEM or TEG should be sent immediately. In the emergency department, patients will likely receive a chest radiograph and electrocardiogram (EKG), particularly if the

Table 2 Management and evaluation of suspected aorto-esophageal fistula	
Resuscitation and Stabilization	Two large-bore IVs Central venous access Arterial line Crystalloid infusion— limited
Airway	Consider intubation if massive hematemesis
Transfusion	Blood and blood products Consider massive transfusion protocol Maintain balanced transfusion Consider IV calcium
Infection Management	Broad-spectrum IV antibiotics IV antifungals
Laboratories	CBC BMP 2 sets of blood cultures Arterial blood gas Coagulation panel (PT/INR) Type and crossmatch TEG or ROTEM
Imaging	Chest radiograph (AP and lateral) CTA chest and abdomen EGD—with caution

Abbreviations: AP, anteroposterior; INR, International Normalized Ratio; PT, prothrombin time.

patient reports ongoing dysphagia or midthoracic pain.

CTA

Computed tomography angiography (CTA) is critical for diagnosis and operative planning for AEF. It offers a high-resolution view of the aorta and associated blood vessels, which provides essential information to assess feasibility of endovascular repair, the need for full or partial cardiopulmonary bypass (CPB), and surgical approach for exposure. CTA can also provide information on aortic pseudoaneurysm, mediastinitis, the extent of any soft tissue involvement, periaortic fluid collections, esophageal or bronchial wall thickening, thoracic contamination, or a new mediastinal mass to suggest contained aortic rupture.[26,34]

For diagnosing AEF, the reported sensitivity ranges from 40% to 93%, and reported specificity ranges from 33% to 100%.[35,36] Imaging mimics of AEF include retroperitoneal fibrosis, infected aortic aneurysms, infectious aortitis, and perigraft infection without fistulization.[36] Differentiation is aided by the observation of highly suggestive features that include ectopic peri-aortic gas, loss of the normal fat plane, extravasation of aortic contrast material into the enteric lumen, or leakage of enteric contrast material into the paraprosthetic space.[36]

EGD

The role of esophagogastroduodenoscopy (EGD) in AEF has been debated, but depending on the patient's history and symptoms, EGD may be a natural step in the workup of an undifferentiated UGIB and can exclude other more common causes of bleeding. For AEF, the reported sensitivity of EGD is lower than CTA, with a reported sensitivity of 25% to 80%.[4,37]

Endoscopic findings of AEF may include visible aortic graft material, pulsatile arterial bleeding, adherent clot, hematoma, esophageal tear, or a pulsatile mass in the esophagus.[27,38,39] The esophageal mucosa may appear blue–gray as a result of submucosal hematoma.[12,38–40] If the patient presents during a period of large-volume hematemesis, EGD will be unable to identify a bleeding source or location due to massive arterial hemorrhage in the GI tract. If the patient is evaluated with EGD during the symptom-free interval, failure to diagnose the AEF may occur due to transient clot formation.[38–40]

EGD should be used cautiously in patients with high suspicion of AEF due to risks of clot disruption that can precipitate fatal exsanguination, enlargement of the aortic defect with esophageal manipulation and insufflation, and potential intubation of the aorta through the fistula tract.[41] Consequently, some clinicians recommend against the use of EGD when AEF is highly suspected given the concern for massive hemorrhage. In cases of suspected foreign body ingestion, radiograph and computed tomography (CT) are useful to determine the position of the foreign body. GI endoscopy can be used to localize and remove foreign bodies but again carries the risk of further aortic damage and fatal bleeding.[23]

THERAPEUTIC OPTIONS

As with other highly morbid surgical emergencies, nonoperative management remains an option that can and should be discussed with the patient and family. For AEF, nonoperative management consists of antibiotics, antifungals, proton pump inhibitor and/or octreotide, enteral or parenteral nutrition, and ongoing resuscitation with fluids, blood products, vasopressors, and general supportive measures. Previous reports establish a 100% mortality rate with nonoperative management,[3] and goals of care should be discussed with the patient and family

if this route is pursued. Definitive TEVAR can be offered to patients who refuse open thoracic surgery. Additionally, patients with multiple comorbidities and limited life expectancy are high risk for open repair, and definitive TEVAR may offer a less invasive alternative in these patients to control acute hemorrhage.[42]

If the patient presents with ongoing massive UGIB, immediate lifesaving hemorrhage control can be attempted with a Sengstaken–Blakemore tube (or Minnesota tube) with gastroesophageal balloon tamponade.[2,8] These devices work by applying direct pressure to the mucosal surfaces through inflation of balloons. However, this risks further esophageal perforation and enlargement of the aorto-esophageal defect, aspiration pneumonitis, and bronchoesophageal fistulas and must be placed by experienced providers.

With recent advances in endovascular techniques, TEVAR may be used as a bridge or destination aortic therapy.[14] As a bridging therapy, TEVAR is an endoluminal aortic stent that provides rapid hemodynamic stabilization by controlling bleeding from the fistula site and thus reducing the risk of sudden life-threatening hematemesis and subsequent circulatory collapse. As a destination aortic therapy, TEVAR does not treat the esophageal disease or esophageal wall defect. It does not address contamination and any ongoing infection conditions in the aorta, thoracic cavity, or mediastinum. TEVAR risks subsequent graft infection, AEF recurrence, fistula re-hemorrhage, mediastinitis, stroke and other neurologic complications, sepsis, and death. Consequently, the consensus is that TEVAR should be performed as a bridging treatment before definitive open aortic surgery or management of the esophageal defect.

Table 3 provides a summary of therapeutic approaches to AEF.

SURGICAL TECHNIQUES

There is considerable variation and lack of standardization in the approach to surgical management of AEF. Given the rarity of the condition, the range of clinical severity, the need for emergent/urgent hemorrhage control, and ongoing advancements in therapeutic options, there is no clear consensus on the ideal operative approach. Much of the available data are based on case reports or small case series, and publication bias (ie, preferentially publishing successful outcomes) may influence available data. Further, the choice of operative approach may vary based on the etiology of the AEF (ie, due to underlying aortic defect vs foreign body ingestion vs malignancy vs iatrogenic/status post-TEVAR). The timing of

Table 3
Therapeutic approach to aorto-esophageal fistula

Massive Hemorrhage	Consider Sengstaken–Blakemore tube or Minnesota tube
TEVAR	Bridging therapy—recommended Definitive aortic therapy
Aortic Defect	Resect/repair—Dacron, Gore-Tex, PTFE, bovine patch Extra-anatomic bypass—select conditions, use with caution Cardiopulmonary bypass—fem/fem or left heart bypass
Esophageal Defect	Primary repair—limited role Esophagectomy with cervical esophagostomy T-tube Esophageal stent—not recommended
Gastrointestinal Reconstruction	Gastric conduit Colonic interposition
Buttress	Omentum Intercostal muscle flap Pleura, adventitia
Thoracic Drainage	Chest tube
Nutritional Access	Total parenteral nutrition Feeding tube—gastrostomy, jejunostomy

repair for the aortic and esophageal defects may be concurrent or staged. The continuity of the GI tract may be restored at the initial operation or during a subsequent operation. In this section, we will review the various operative approaches and surgical techniques available for the management of AEF.

General Principles

With operative intervention on AEF, there must be consideration of the aortic defect, the esophageal defect, and mediastinal contamination. While TEVAR allows for acute hemorrhage control, open thoracic surgery allows for repair of the involved aortic and esophageal components of the fistula, as well as irrigation and drainage of the infected mediastinum.

Left posterolateral thoracotomy is the most frequently used approach to gain exposure to the aorta and esophagus.[43] The patient is positioned in a right lateral decubitus position, and a posterolateral skin incision is made from the anterior axillary line to the subscapular area.[43] The left pleural cavity is entered through the fourth or fifth intercostal space, and the chest is opened. An intercostal muscle flap may be harvested during entry if there is a need for a vascularized muscle interposition between the aortic and esophageal defect. After heparinization and establishment of partial or total CPB, aortic control is achieved proximally at the arch and distally at the lower descending aorta.[43] The aorta is then incised and back bleeding from intercostals is controlled. The fistula is identified,

and any aneurysm sac is resected. Surrounding necrotic tissue should be debrided. A vascular graft is then sutured in place to restore aortic continuity.

Management of the esophageal defect consists of either takedown of the fistula with primary repair or esophageal diversion via esophagectomy. Esophagectomy is performed while maintaining lower body perfusion, and the proximal and distal ends of the esophagus are closed with a tissue stapler temporarily. The pleural cavity should be debrided and copiously irrigated. After termination of CPB, a pedicled omental buttress should be brought through the diaphragm into the left pleural cavity and wrapped around the aortic graft.[44] Omental tissue has been used in the management of surgical infection because of its high vascularity and neovascularization potential, leading to a good oxygen supply and an enhanced immune reaction in the infected area.[44] The proximal stump of the esophagus is brought up to the left neck and a cervical esophagostomy is made below the clavicle onto the anterior chest wall. A gastrostomy and jejunostomy are also made for nutrition purposes as restoration of continuity is not made for 3 to 6 months following the procedure.

Approach to the Aortic Defect

For initial stabilization and rapid hemorrhage control, TEVAR is recommended as a damage-control procedure for bridging to aortic graft replacement and definitive repair.[35] While it has been proposed by some as an alternative to surgical intervention,[45–47] TEVAR presents important limitations in treating AEF, primarily due to graft infection via unrepaired fistula, ongoing mediastinal contamination, and the subsequent risks of sepsis, re-fistulization, and re-hemorrhage.[13]

A TEVAR-alone strategy has demonstrated poor mid-term and long-term outcomes.[42,45,48] Survival is significantly better after bridging TEVAR followed by aortic graft replacement than after definitive TEVAR, which did not improve survival rates at 6 or 18 months after surgery.[47,49] Consequently, TEVAR is recommended for initial hemorrhage control that bridges to a definitive open aortic surgery.

For definitive aortic surgery, primary repair and aortic graft replacement are 2 options. Primary repair of the aorta has been reported in small case series, but this is usually only feasible after a limited injury that occurs from an insult such as a swallowed foreign body.[6,50] The reports after primary aortic repair are limited and largely unsuccessful, and we therefore conditionally recommend against primary aortic repair.

Aortic graft replacement is considered the definitive open aortic repair. There is no consensus on optimal aortic substitute and various options may be unavailable at certain centers. Material of choice for aortic replacement includes Dacron graft, with or without antibiotic treatment (eg, rifampicin), Gore-Tex graft, polytetraflouroethylene (PTFE) graft, and cryopreserved aortic allograft.[51–53] Alternatively, orthotopic aortic reconstruction via bovine pericardial patch as a neoartoa has been described in the literature.[28,54–56] A simple continuous or interrupted technique with a 4-0 or 3-0 monofilament suture with felt reinforcement may be used for anastomosis.

When available, CPB allows for safer and more reliable aortic surgery, enabling resection of involved aorta and implantation of the vascular prosthesis. Partial bypass may be used when clamping the aorta at the aortic arch; if an aortic arch replacement is required, total CPB is recommended. Antegrade cerebral perfusion can be used for patients undergoing aortic arch reconstruction. The proximal and distal ends of the descending aorta may be cross-clamped, the aorta incised, back bleeding from intercostal arteries controlled with sutures. The fistula should be identified, and the aneurysm sac resected as much as possible. Surrounding necrotic tissue should be debrided. The vascular prosthesis is anastomosed to a healthy aorta.

The Role of Extra-anatomic Bypass

Extra-anatomic bypass (EAB) has been proposed as an alternative to in situ aortic graft replacement to prevent secondary graft infection from mediastinal contamination, and it has been advocated in cases of severe mediastinal sepsis.[55,57,58] The EAB has been performed from the ascending aorta to the abdominal aorta (supraceliac and infrarenal) or axillary to the bilateral femoral arteries. However, these procedures carry significant morbidity, including late rupture of the aortic stump and risks for inadequate perfusion of the lower body.[57]

Approach to Esophageal Defect

The esophageal defect has been managed through a variety of surgical approaches. Options for esophageal management include direct suture repair, patch repair, T tube intubation, partial or total esophagectomy, or esophageal stenting.[47,53,57,59,60] The timing of esophageal management and subsequent reconstruction can be concurrent with aortic surgery or staged in a secondary surgery.

When performed concurrently with open aortic surgery, direct suture repair or esophageal resection with immediate esophagogastroplasty or coloplasty has been reported as viable options.[14,47] However, direct suture repair has a limited role. It has been reported as an option when the esophageal defect is small, the surrounding esophageal walls are without necrosis, and there is no gross contamination.[47] Consequently, direct suture repair is not applicable to many AEF scenarios, particularly those with significant esophageal injury, tissue damage, or mediastinal infection. A second option for concurrent repair includes esophagectomy and immediate reconstruction with esophagogastroplasty or coloplasty. Advantages of esophagectomy include definitive management of the fistula and decreased risk of aortic graft contamination from the esophagus. A drawback of esophagectomy is the loss of alimentary continuity and the need for delayed reconstruction. If patients have had previous abdominal operations, specifically gastric procedures, conduit options for restoration of continuity may be limited. Esophageal stenting can be used as a temporary measure while a definitive esophageal procedure is being planned. Esophageal stenting is contraindicated in patients undergoing TEVAR as the 2 adjacent stents can lead to worsening fistula, further esophageal necrosis or TEVAR stent infection. Esophageal stenting has a reported 17% 1 year survival rate and is not widely supported for management of the esophageal injury.[61] A staged approach to the esophageal defect has the best prognosis and has been advocated in the literature. This approach consists of an initial esophagectomy with cervical esophagostomy (performed after aortic repair under CPB with distal perfusion maintained via femoro-femoral

CPB), concomitant gastrostomy, or jejunostomy, followed by a period of nutritional optimization and infection management, with postponed esophageal reconstruction.[53,59,60] Reconstruction of the GI continuity may consist of either a cervical esophagogastrostomy or pedicled colon interposition through a substernal or ante-sternal route.[53] Timing of the delayed reconstruction has been reported from 1 to 3 months after the initial operation.

CONTROVERSIES AND DISCUSSION

AEF is a challenging clinical entity. The first challenge occurs with patient presentation, which may vary widely from vague dysphagia and midthoracic back pain, to undifferentiated shock, to fatal hemorrhage. With this spectrum of presenting symptoms, maintaining AEF on the differential diagnosis is paramount. EGD, the classic tool for diagnosing, localizing, and treating an acute UGIB, may precipitate fatal hemorrhage in patients with AEF through clot disruption or accidental intubation of the aorta through the fistula tract.

The challenges and controversies do not stop once the diagnosis is made. No clear consensus exists for the optimal surgical management of this diagnosis, and the choice of management may vary based on etiology, acuity, and clinical status. Some advocate for definitive TEVAR, some advocate for concurrent definitive aortic and esophageal management, and others advocate for a staged approach to esophageal management and reconstruction.

While controversy exists, there is strong evidence against certain approaches. We know that nonoperative approaches result in 100% 1 year mortality.[3] Data are clear that TEVAR alone does not provide a complete and durable cure for AEF, and these patients must be followed closely to evaluate the opportunity and appropriate timing for a secondary surgical esophageal and aortic procedure. There is no general consensus concerning the need or timing for planned staged surgical intervention following the successful use of TEVAR in the absence of clear signs of reinfection or bleeding. A recent multicenter report analyzing patients with AEF who underwent TEVAR-alone found that there were no 1 year survivors without esophagectomy.[18] Large reviews have demonstrated that the combination of aortic graft replacement, radical esophagectomy, and omental buttress has the most favorable prognosis of all therapies.[14,18]

COMPLICATIONS/CONCERNS

Prompt diagnosis and emergent surgery are necessary but not sufficient for the survival of AEF. Even with rapid management, mortality remains high risk postoperatively. Sepsis and re-hemorrhage are primary causes of death postoperatively, as AEF is essentially an infection in which the bacteria-free aorta becomes contaminated by material from the GI tract. Postoperatively, these complications may be attributable to the infection of the aortic graft caused by mediastinal contamination or remnant infection from the preexisting fistula tract. Postoperative death has been reported from mediastinitis, multi-organ failure, and fatal bleeding from erosion of adjacent anatomic structures. Given the high reports (>50%) of patients dying from sepsis after surgery, recommendations have been made for lifelong suppressive antibiotics.[14,35] Many centers advocate for ongoing clinical and imaging follow-up with standard protocols for postoperative CT scans at 1, 3, 6, and 12 months and then yearly.[47]

SUMMARY AND FUTURE DIRECTIONS

AEFs are a rare cause of massive GI bleeding and are lethal unless recognized early. Early recognition of clinical symptoms and prompt resuscitation followed by expeditious intervention are key to limiting mortality associated with these fistulas. The mainstay of intervention for primary AEF includes open takedown of the fistula with esophageal repair or diversion followed by aortic repair either primarily or replacement. Success has also been reported utilizing aortic stenting via TEVAR, however, is limited to advanced aortic centers. When placing TEVAR for management of fistulas, esophageal diversion must be considered at the time of primary intervention or at a later time to avoid infection of the graft.

CLINICS CARE POINTS

- AEFs are a rare source of UGIB and a high index of suspicion is imperative for prompt treatment.
- Primary management includes resuscitation involving fluid and blood with CT imaging being the gold standard of diagnosis.
- Once AEF is diagnosed, prompt surgical intervention with fistula exclusion either by open repair or TEVAR is recommended.
- Esophageal repair can be performed at the time of aortic management or can be delayed for a short period of time. Esophageal repair is indicated to avoid aortic graft infection.

DISCLOSURE

Dr L.J. Schoel receives funding from the National Institute on Aging, United States National Research Service Award (T32-AG062403). The authors have no conflicts of interest or disclosures to the work therein.

REFERENCES

1. Zhan Y, Xu Z. Massive hemorrhage from an aortoesophageal fistula caused by esophageal stent implantation: A case report and literature review. Medicine 2019;98(51):e18303.
2. D'Amore K, Swaminathan A. Massive Gastrointestinal Hemorrhage. Emerg Med Clin 2020;38(4):871–89.
3. Hollander JE, Quick G. Aortoesophageal Fistula: A comprehensive review of the literature. Am J Med 1991;91(3):279–87.
4. Saers SJF, Scheltinga MRM. Primary aortoenteric fistula. Br J Surg 2005;92(2):143–52.
5. Dubrueil O. Observations sur la perforation de l'esophage et de l'aorte thoracique par une portion d'os avale: avec de reflexions. J Univ Sci Med 1818;9:357–63.
6. Ctercteko G, Mok CK. Aorta-esophageal fistula induced by a foreign body: the first recorded survival. J Thorac Cardiovasc Surg 1980;80(2):233–5.
7. Nandi P, Ong GB. Foreign body in the oesophagus: Review of 2394 cases. Br J Surg 2005;65(1):5–9.
8. Carter R, Mulder GA, Snyder EN, et al. Aortoesophageal fistula. Am J Surg 1978;136(1):26–30.
9. Katyal D, Jewell LD, Yakimets WW. Aorto-esophageal fistula secondary to benign Barrett's ulcer: a rare cause of massive gastrointestinal hemorrhage. Canadian Journal of Surgery. Journal Canadien De Chirurgie 1993;36(5):480–2.
10. Chiesa R, Melissano G, Marone EM, et al. Aorto-oesophageal and Aortobronchial Fistulae Following Thoracic Endovascular Aortic Repair: A National Survey. Eur J Vasc Endovasc Surg 2010;39(3):273–9.
11. Dossa CD, Pipinos II, Shepard AD, et al. Primary Aortoenteric Fistula: Part I. Ann Vasc Surg 1994; 8(1):113–20.
12. Pipinos II, Reddy DJ. Secondary Aortoesophageal Fistulae. Ann Vasc Surg 1999;13(6):649–52.
13. Mosquera VX, Marini M, Pombo-Felipe F, et al. Predictors of outcome and different management of aortobronchial and aortoesophageal fistulas. J Thorac Cardiovasc Surg 2014;148(6):3020–6.e2.
14. Takeno S, Ishii H, Nanashima A, et al. Aortoesophageal fistula: review of trends in the last decade. Surg Today 2020;50(12):1551–9.
15. Hsu WF, Lin CC, Chang KM, et al. Primary aortoesophageal fistula: A rare but fatal cause of upper gastrointestinal bleeding. Journal of Digestive Diseases 2013;14(12):676–8.
16. Xi E-P, Zhu J, Zhu S-B, et al. Secondary aortoesophageal fistula after thoracic aortic aneurysm endovascular repair: literature review and new insights regarding the hypothesized mechanisms. Int J Clin Exp Med 2014;7(10):3244–52.
17. Isasti G, Gómez-Doblas JJ, Olalla E. Aortoesophageal fistula: an uncommon complication after stent-graft repair of an aortic thoracic aneurysm. Interact Cardiovasc Thorac Surg 2009;9(4):683–4.
18. Czerny M, Eggebrecht H, Sodeck G, et al. New insights regarding the incidence, presentation and treatment options of aorto-oesophageal fistulation after thoracic endovascular aortic repair: the European Registry of Endovascular Aortic Repair Complications. Eur J Cardio Thorac Surg 2014;45(3): 452–7.
19. Chiesa R, Melissano G, Marone EM, et al. Endovascular treatment of aortoesophageal and aortobronchial fistulae. J Vasc Surg 2010;51(5):1195–202.
20. Eggebrecht H, Mehta RH, Dechene A, et al. Aortoesophageal Fistula After Thoracic Aortic Stent-Graft Placement. JACC Cardiovasc Interv 2009;2(6): 570–6.
21. Albors J, Ángel Bahamonde J, Manuel Sanchis J, et al. Aortoesophageal fistula after thoracic stent grafting. Asian Cardiovasc Thorac Ann 2011;19(5): 352–6.
22. Li S. [Aorto-esophageal fistula caused by swallowed foreign body (report of 17 cases)]. Zhonghua Er Bi Yan Hou Ke Za Zhi 1992;27(2):91–2, 125–126.
23. Wei Y, Chen L, Wang Y, et al. Proposed management protocol for ingested esophageal foreign body and aortoesophageal fistula: a single-center experience. Int J Clin Exp Med 2015;8(1):607–15.
24. Zhang X, Liu J, Li J, et al. Diagnosis and treatment of 32 cases with aortoesophageal fistula due to esophageal foreign body. Laryngoscope 2011;121(2): 267–72.
25. Lai ATY, Chow TL, Lee DTY, et al. Risk factors predicting the development of complications after foreign body ingestion. Br J Surg 2003;90(12):1531–5.
26. Kieffer E, Chiche L, Gomes D. Aortoesophageal Fistula: Value of In Situ Aortic Allograft Replacement. Ann Surg 2003;238(2):283–90.
27. Heckstall RL, Hollander JE. Aortoesophageal Fistula: Recognition and Diagnosis in the Emergency Department. Ann Emerg Med 1998;32(4):502–5.
28. Al-Thani H, Wahlen BM, El-Menyar A, et al. Presentation, management and outcome of aorto-esophageal fistula in young patients: two case-reports and literature review. J Surg Case Rep 2021;2021(6):rjab213.
29. Sica GS, Djapardy V, Westaby S, et al. Diagnosis and management of aortoesophageal fistula caused by a foreign body. Ann Thorac Surg 2004;77(6):2217–8.
30. Villanueva C, Colomo A, Bosch A, et al. Transfusion strategies for acute upper gastrointestinal bleeding. N Engl J Med 2013;368(1):11–21.

31. Ley EJ, Clond MA, Srour MK, et al. Emergency department crystalloid resuscitation of 1.5 l or more is associated with increased mortality in elderly and nonelderly trauma patients. J Trauma Inj Infect Crit Care 2011;70(2):398–400.

32. Kaczynski J, Wilczynska M, Hilton J, et al. Impact of crystalloids and colloids on coagulation cascade during trauma resuscitation-a literature review. Emerg Med Health Care 2013;1(1):1.

33. Hans GA, Besser MW. The place of viscoelastic testing in clinical practice. Br J Haematol 2016; 173(1):37–48.

34. Tierney LM, Wall SD, Jacobs RA. Aortoesophageal fistula after perigraft abscess with characteristic CT Findings. J Clin Gastroenterol 1984;6(6):535–7.

35. Baril DT, Carroccio A, Ellozy SH, et al. Evolving strategies for the treatment of aortoenteric fistulas. J Vasc Surg 2006;44(2):250–7.

36. Vu QDM, Menias CO, Bhalla S, et al. Aortoenteric Fistulas: CT Features and Potential Mimics. Radiographics 2009;29(1):197–209.

37. Champion MC, Sullivan SN, Coles JC, et al. Aortoenteric fistula: incidence, presentation recognition, and management. Ann Surg 1982;195(3):314–7.

38. Khawaja FI, Varindani MK. Review of clinical, radiographic, and endoscopic features. J Clin Gastroenterol 1987;9(3):342–4.

39. Kirchgatterer A, Punzengruber C, Zisch R, et al. A rare case of gastrointestinal hemorrhage: aortoesophageal fistula following repair of aortic dissection. Endoscopy 1997;29(02):137–8.

40. Sinar DR, DeMaria A, Kataria YP, et al. Aortic aneurysm eroding the esophagus case report and review. Am J Dig Dis 1977;22(3):252–4.

41. Fukunaga N, Matsueda T, Osumi M, et al. Unexpectedly large aortoesophageal fistula inconsistent with CT imaging due to the thrombus working as the tamponade. J Cardiol 2009;54(3):466–9.

42. Burks JA, Faries PL, Gravereaux EC, et al. Endovascular repair of bleeding aortoenteric fistulas: A 5-year experience. J Vasc Surg 2001;34(6):1055–9.

43. Yamazato T, Nakamura T, Abe N, et al. Surgical strategy for the treatment of aortoesophageal fistula. J Thorac Cardiovasc Surg 2018;155(1):32–40.

44. Kitayama J, Morota T, Kaisaki S, et al. Complete coverage of in situ aortograft by total omental pedicle flap as the most reliable treatment of aortoesophageal fistula. Am J Surg 2006;192(1):130–4.

45. Léobon B, Roux D, Mugniot A, et al. Endovascular treatment of thoracic aortic fistulas. Ann Thorac Surg 2002;74(1):247–9.

46. Taylor BJW, Stewart D, West P, et al. Endovascular Repair of a Secondary Aortoesophageal Fistula: a Case Report and Review of the Literature. Ann Vasc Surg 2007;21(2):167–71.

47. Marone EM, Coppi G, Kahlberg A, et al. Combined endovascular and surgical treatment of primary aortoesophageal fistula. Tex Heart Inst J 2010; 37(6):722–4.

48. González-Fajardo JA, Gutiérrez V, Martín-Pedrosa M, et al. Endovascular Repair in the Presence of Aortic Infection. Ann Vasc Surg 2005;19(1):94–8.

49. Akashi H, Kawamoto S, Saiki Y, et al. Therapeutic strategy for treating aortoesophageal fistulas. General Thoracic and Cardiovascular Surgery 2014; 62(10):573–80.

50. Snyder DM, Crawford ES. Successful treatment of primary aorta-esophageal fistula resulting from aortic aneurysm. J Thorac Cardiovasc Surg 1983; 85(3):457–63.

51. Fatima J, Duncan AA, De Grandis E, et al. Treatment strategies and outcomes in patients with infected aortic endografts. J Vasc Surg 2013;58(2):371–9.

52. Vogt PR, Brunner-LaRocca H-P, Lachat M, et al. Technical details with the use of cryopreserved arterial allografts for aortic infection: Influence on early and midterm mortality. J Vasc Surg 2002;35(1):80–6.

53. Okita Y, Yamanaka K, Okada K, et al. Strategies for the treatment of aorto-oesophageal fistula. Eur J Cardio Thorac Surg 2014;46(5):894–900.

54. Czerny M, Zimpfer D, Fleck T, et al. Successful Treatment of an Aortoesophageal Fistula After Emergency Endovascular Thoracic Aortic Stent-Graft Placement. Ann Thorac Surg 2005;80(3):1117–20.

55. Topel I, Stehr A, Steinbauer MG, et al. Surgical Strategy in Aortoesophageal Fistulae: Endovascular Stentgrafts and In Situ Repair of the Aorta With Cryopreserved Homografts. Ann Surg 2007;246(5): 853–9.

56. Hwang SH, Cho JW, Bae CH, et al. Staged Surgical Treatment of Primary Aortoesophageal Fistula. The Korean Journal of Thoracic and Cardiovascular Surgery 2019;52(3):182–5.

57. Madan AK, Santora TA, DiSesa VJ. Extra-anatomic bypass grafting for aortoesophageal fistula: A logical operation. J Vasc Surg 2000;32(5):1030–3.

58. Prokakis C, Koletsis E, Apostolakis E, et al. Aortoesophageal fistulas due to thoracic aorta aneurysm: surgical versus endovascular repair. Is there a role for combined aortic management? Med Sci Mon Int Med J Exp Clin Res: International Medical Journal of Experimental and Clinical Research 2008; 14(4):RA48–54.

59. Tkebuchava T, Von Segesser LK, Turina MI. Successful Repair of Primary Concomitant Aortobronchial and Aortoesophageal Fistulas. Ann Thorac Surg 1997;63(6):1779–81.

60. Kubota S, Shiiya N, Shingu Y, et al. Surgical strategy for aortoesophageal fistula in the endovascular era. General Thoracic and Cardiovascular Surgery 2013; 61(10):560–4.

61. Dumfarth J, Dejaco H, Krapf C, et al. Aorto-Esophageal Fistula After Thoracic Endovascular Aortic Repair: Successful Open Treatment. AORTA 2014;2(1):37–40.

Esophageal-Pericardial and Esophageal-Atrial Fistulae

Jacqueline M. Soegaard Ballester, MD, MBMI*, John C. Kucharczuk, MD

KEYWORDS

- Esophageal-pericardial fistula • Esophageal-atrial fistula • Atrial-esophageal fistula
- Esophageal fistula • Catheter-based ablation complications

KEY POINTS

- Fistulae between the esophagus and the pericardium or the left atrium are rare but feared complications of transcatheter ablations and esophageal procedures and pathologies.
- Patients may present variably with cardiopulmonary, gastrointestinal, infectious, and/or neurologic symptoms; a high index of suspicion is paramount to enable timely diagnosis, stabilization, and treatment.
- While mortality is high overall, surgical repair confers the highest likelihood of survival. Other endoscopic or nonsurgical drainage procedures have been reported.
- The presence of atrial involvement will dictate the approach and extent of the necessary intervention.

INTRODUCTION

Fistulae between the esophagus and the pericardium or the left atrium are rare but feared, and often fatal, complications of cardiac and esophageal procedures and pathologies. Given the emergent nature and relative infrequency of esophageal-pericadial fistulae (EPF) or esophageal-atrial fistulae (EAF), our understanding of these disease processes stems largely from case series and reports. A high index of suspicion and early identification are paramount if successful treatment is to be attempted prior to catastrophic neurologic or hemorrhagic complications. Different treatment strategies and sequences have been suggested, but optimal treatment should be individualized.

NATURE OF THE PROBLEM

As with other types of fistulous connections in the body, EPF and EAF may arise from a wide-ranging series of insults or contexts that create a favorable milieu for fistula formation. These may include direct injury (either mechanical or thermal), chronic inflammation or infection, radiation, neoplastic growth, and distal obstruction.[1] While both are morbid conditions that are challenging to manage clinically and operatively, the limited data available suggest that EAFs carry a higher mortality than EPFs.[2] In early reports, most cases stemmed from chronic esophageal pathologies, such as chronic gastroesophageal reflux with esophagitis, strictures, ulcers, Barrett's esophagus, and hiatal hernias.[3,4] Other reported causes include advanced achalasia, caustic ingestions, and radiation-induced esophagitis.[5,6] Locally advanced esophageal malignancies may directly invade the pericardium, leading to primary fistula formation.[7–11] Prior esophageal dilations, surgeries, or resections, particularly those complicated by leaks, may also result in these fistulae.[12–15] More recently, transcatheter ablation procedures for atrial arrhythmias and esophageal

Department of Surgery, Hospital of the University of Pennsylvania, 3400 Spruce Street, 4th Floor Silverstein, Philadelphia, PA 19104, USA
* Corresponding author. Department of Surgery, Hospital of the University of Pennsylvania, 4th Floor Silverstein, 3400 Spruce Street, Philadelphia, PA 19104.
E-mail address: Jacqueline.Soegaard@pennmedicine.upenn.edu

Thorac Surg Clin 34 (2024) 395–403
https://doi.org/10.1016/j.thorsurg.2024.05.003
1547-4127/24/© 2024 Elsevier Inc. All rights are reserved, including those for text and data mining, AI training, and similar technologies.

stents have also arisen as an iatrogenic causes of EAF.[2]

While rare, EAFs between the posterior wall of the left atrium and the esophagus have become an increasingly common complication of surgical and catheter-based ablation procedures for atrial fibrillation and other arrhythmias. The mechanism for esophageal perforation or fistulization after these procedures has been postulated to be due to direct thermal injury causing an inflammatory response in the esophageal wall, or to thermal injury to the esophageal arteries coursing anterior to the esophagus causing ischemia and necrosis of the esophageal wall.[16] Damage to vagal fibers resulting in impaired lower esophageal sphincter function and increased reflux may also contribute and exacerbate mucosal injury.[17,18] Routine endoscopic surveillance after ablation procedures has identified esophageal injuries and ulcerations in about 15% to 20% of patients, although studies report a wide range of incidence estimates, some much higher.[19,20] While most heal, in some cases these sentinel injuries can progress to deep ulcers and fistulae. In one study, patients followed with routine post-procedure endoscopy were found to have a 9.6% risk of progression from ulcer to fistula or perforation.[20]

Estimates of the incidence of EAF after ablation procedures have ranged between from 0.015% to 0.25%.[19,21–23] More recently, the POTTER-AF trial, an international multicenter registry study across 214 centers in 35 countries, quantified the risk of EAF after catheter ablation procedures as 0.025% (n = 138/553,729).[2] Among patients for whom complete peri-procedural data were available (n = 118/138), the incidence of fistula was significantly lower for cryoballoon ablation (0.0015%) than for radiofrequency ablation (0.038%). The median time to symptoms was 18 days following the ablation, with fever being the most common presenting symptom (59.3%), followed by chest pain or odynophagia (54.2%), and neurologic signs (44.1%). Notably, the median time from symptom onset to fistula diagnosis was 3 days.

Esophageal stenting, which has become a commonly-used strategy to address esophageal perforations and strictures, as well as a palliative strategy for obstructing esophageal tumors, also carry a risk of fistulization between the esophagus and surrounding structures such as the pericardium or the airway.[24,25] The radial force these stents generate can lead to erosion and fistulization over time, particularly when used amidst a backdrop of surrounding cancerous tissue (which in some cases has been further weakened by systemic and radiation therapies). Surgeons and

proceduralists utilizing such stents should remain vigilant for this complication.

ANATOMY

The posterior wall of the left atrium closely abuts the mid thoracic esophagus, which is defined as the region of esophagus between the carinal bifurcation and the inferior pulmonary veins, about 25–30 cm from the incisors. Beyond the pericardium, a fibroadipose plane between these 2 structures contains lymph nodes, branches of the left vagus nerves, and esophageal arteries arising from the descending thoracic aorta. The position and angle of the esophagus relative to the left atrial structures can both be anatomically variable amongst individuals (and may be affected by displacement from the descending thoracic aorta), and also may vary with time given the relative mobility of the esophagus.

Cadaveric studies have shed light on the relationships between these structures.[16] The area of esophagus in contact with the posterior left atrial wall is approximately 42 ± 7 mm in length and 13.5 ± 5 mm in width. There is significant variation in the distance between the endocardium and the esophageal wall, ranging from 3.3 to 13.5 mm, with 40% of examined specimens having a distance less than 5 mm. This distance is not uniform across the entire area of contact, which relates to the variable thickness of the posterior left atrial wall as well as the fibroadipose plane between the atrium and the esophagus. The posterior left atrial wall is thinner more superiorly and becomes thicker more inferiorly closer to the mitral annulus. The thickness of the atrial wall is also lowest more laterally next to the pulmonary vein orifices, and thickest in the midpoint of the posterior atrial wall. In contrast, the fibroadipose plane between the atrium and the esophagus is thickest superiorly, and thinnest inferiorly at the level of the inferior pulmonary veins.

PREVENTION

Several preventive techniques have been proposed to reduce the risk of EAF after atrial ablation procedures.[19,26] Consensus on the best protective approaches is lacking given the quality of the evidence. Given the inherent challenges in studying the prevention of such a rare complication as EAF or EPF, these data are largely based on studies that assessed for differences in rates of esophageal thermal injury or ulceration.

Most interventionalists will administer postprocedural acid suppression with proton pump inhibitors or H2 blockers, albeit without clear data to support this practice.[17] Since higher esophageal temperatures are associated with higher rates of injury, the use of continuous esophageal temperature monitoring has been recommended.[18] This theoretically enables operators to avoid exceeding safe temperatures, although results have been variable across studies and there is no consensus on the optimal temperature threshold values. It is also recommended to decrease the power when applying energy to the posterior left atrial wall, which is in closest proximity with the esophagus. Esophageal cooling devices have also been proposed, and a recent multicenter study has demonstrated promising results.[18,27]

The case-specific anatomic relationships are also important for procedural planning. Axial imaging can aid in understanding the relative position of the esophagus and the left atrium, since the risk of esophageal injury increases as this distance gets shorter. Beyond pre-procedural planning, real-time identification of the esophageal position relative to the left atrium with various adjunctive technologies has been suggested as a way to avoid application of power in the most vulnerable regions.[26] In cases when the distance is short, the use of devices to displace the esophagus away from the left atrium has been reported.[18,28]

The choice of anesthesia may also affect rates of esophageal tissue damage. One study identified significantly lower rates of post-ablation tissue damage in patients undergoing ablation under conscious sedation as opposed to general anesthesia (4% vs 48%, $P<.001$).[29] This was likely related to the higher maximal esophageal temperatures and faster time to peak temperature observed in the general anesthesia cohort.

Some experts advocate for routine endoluminal surveillance of the esophagus after ablation procedures via conventional or capsule endoscopy.[20,29,30] This can permit identification of areas of thermal injury or early ulceration that may be at high risk for progression to a fistula. For such sentinel lesions, patients can first be treated with supportive measures—including enteral nutrition, sublingual atropine to reduce salivary secretions, proton pump inhibitors, and sucralfate—and should be followed with close monitoring and surveilled with repeat endoscopy. For ulcers demonstrating endoscopic progression, the successful use of endoclip techniques or of endoluminal negative pressure vacuum therapy for treatment of earlier-stage esophageal ulcers after ablation procedures has been reported and may be considered.[30,31]

CLINICAL PRESENTATION

Patients with EAF and EPF may present with a constellation of clinical findings spanning cardiac,

pulmonary, esophageal, infectious, and neurologic symptoms (**Table 1**).[2,7,8,32–41] These symptoms stem from sequelae of inflammation or mediastinitis, accumulation of fluid in the pericardial or pleural spaces, entrainment of air or esophageal particulate matter into the circulation, and bleeding. In particular, small fistulae may permit the passage of air and bacteria without more obvious passage of fluid or blood.[25]

Patients may present with these symptoms while under the care of cardiac or thoracic specialists, or may present in an emergency setting where the initial evaluation is guided by a non-specialist. Careful attention to symptomatology and recent procedural history are essential for raising the possibility of EAF or EPF. Physical examination may be initially unrevealing, except for the case of obvious neurologic deficits.

In the atrial fibrillation population, it is important to consider that thromboembolic strokes are a much more common etiology for neurologic infarction symptoms.[19] Therefore, a careful attention to recent procedural history is important to establish whether an antecedent radiofrequency ablation

Table 1
Presenting symptoms associated with esophageal-atrial or esophageal-pericardial fistulae

System	Symptoms
Cardiopulmonary	Atypical chest pain Substernal chest pain Pleuritic chest pain Dyspnea Cough Syncope
Gastrointestinal	Nausea Vomiting Dysphagia Odynophagia Heartburn Hematemesis Melena Occult blood in stool
Constitutional/ Infectious	Fever Chills Malaise
Neurologic	Monocular blindness Facial droop Hemiparesis Aphasia Seizure Headache Altered consciousness or confusion Hyperreflexia

was performed that introduces EAF fistula as a possible alternate etiology for neurologic symptoms.

DIAGNOSTIC EVALUATION

Given the heterogeneous possible presentations, initial diagnostic imaging is often determined by initial presenting symptoms. These early imaging modalities may range from plain chest radiographs to transthoracic echocardiograms, chest computed tomography, and others. While nonspecific, in the right clinical context, the imaging signs noted in **Table 2** should raise suspicion for a possible esophageal-pericardial or esophageal-atrial fistula and should prompt further investigation and close patient monitoring. In the POTTER-AF study, chest computed tomography was used in 80.2% of the cases, although often multiple modalities were used to establish the diagnosis.[2] Maintaining a high index of suspicion is paramount given that initial axial imaging may not demonstrate an obvious communication.[42]

Pericardial effusions or esophageal thermal injuries after ablation procedures may be sentinel signs, and should prompt further evaluation to rule out an EAF. This may facilitate earlier diagnosis prior to esophageal injury progressing to frank perforation and mediastinal contamination, with the ensuing impact on tissue quality for primary esophageal repair.

PREOPERATIVE STABILIZATION AND PLANNING

In preparing for intervention to correct these fistulae, the following considerations should be addressed.

- *Intravenous antimicrobial therapy:* Patients should be immediately started and maintained on broad-spectrum intravenous antimicrobial therapy with activity against gram negative, anaerobic, and fungal organisms.
- *Neurologic stabilization:* Patients presenting with symptoms of cerebrovascular accident as part of their symptomatology should have prompt consultation with a stroke neurology team. Decisions for subsequent interventions should be performed in conjunction with the stroke team to triage and balance concurrent urgent patient issues.
- *Cardiopulmonary support and drainage:* Patients should receive immediate and adequate cardiopulmonary critical care with endotracheal intubation, mechanical ventilation, invasive monitoring, resuscitation, and vasopressor

Table 2 Imaging findings that may raise suspicion for esophageal-atrial or esophageal-pericardial fistulae	
Study	**Findings**
Chest radiograph	Pleural effusion or hydropneumothorax Pneumomediastinum or hydropneumomediastinum Enlarged cardiac silhouette or mediastinal widening
Transthoracic echocardiogram	Pericardial effusion, pneumopericardium, or hydropneumopericardium Tamponade physiology Intracardiac air Flow through atrial defect
Chest computed tomography	Pleural effusion or hydropneumothorax Pneumomediastinum or hydropneumomediastinum Pericardial effusion, pneumopericardium, or hydropneumopericardium IV contrast extravasation from atria PO contrast extravasation from the esophagus Esophageal thickening Fat stranding between the left atrium/pericardium and the esophagus
Contrast esophagogram	Oral contrast extravasation from the esophagus
Brain axial imaging (computed tomography or MRI)	Cerebral air emboli Cerebral infarction
Esophagogastroduodenoscopy	Inflammation or dimpling Endoluminal blood Fistula tract Ulcer

support as needed and appropriate. Although wider drainage will also be accomplished during operative repair of these fistulae, hydropneumothoraces should be drained as soon as possible, particularly if causing cardiopulmonary compromise. The same is true of hydropneumopericardium or pericardial effusion with tamponade physiology. Early drainage is particularly important in cases where nonoperative strategies are being considered, particularly if endoscopic approaches are being considered, since insufflation during endoscopy may cause pneumopericardium or tension pneumothorax.[24]

- *Acid suppression:* Patients should be initiated on proton pump inhibitor or H2 blocker therapy for acid suppression.
- *Nutrition:* Patients will likely face extended *nil per os* status, and nutritional optimization should be considered from the outset to optimize healing. Given that nasoenteric feeding tubes should not be utilized in this population, in the absence of an existing gastrostomy or jejunostomy tube, early initiation of parenteral nutrition should be considered once the patient has been appropriately stabilized.

Patients presenting to hospitals without the necessary cardiac, thoracic, or critical care capabilities should be stabilized and promptly transferred to specialized centers for care. Frank conversations should be had with the patient and their decision makers regarding the high morbidity and mortality of this condition. Such discussions will help set expectations and facilitate decision-making that aligns with the patient's goals of care.

SURGICAL APPROACHES

While all EPFs and EAFs should be addressed urgently, the presence of an EAF with possibility of air entrainment into the arterial circulation or hemorrhage are surgical emergencies that should be immediately addressed. The presence of atrial involvement will also dictate the extent of the necessary intervention. Given the rarity of this condition, our understanding of surgical approaches stems from case series and reports, and from the management of similar pathologies such as esophageal perforations. Of note, many case reports describe repairs of AEF resulting from ablation procedures. Fistulae arising in the setting of prior esophagectomy or other esophageal surgery, neoplastic growth, or as a result of an esophageal stent may pose additional operative challenges.

Esophageal-Pericardial Fistulae

Isolated EPFs without atrial involvement may be approached through a right thoracic approach, either a posterolateral thoracotomy or thoracoscopy as the clinical situation allows. In these scenarios, drainage of the pericardial space by creating a pericardial window and placing surgical drains is essential. The location of the fistula should be identified if possible. When identification is challenging, upper endoscopy or intraoperative esophageal administration of a visual agent to identify location of fistula (methylene blue) may be considered.[15] The esophageal injury and fistula can be repaired primarily at the index operation. This should be done in 2 layers and may be buttressed with an intercostal muscle flap or other tissue flap. The esophageal defect may also be addressed with conservative measures such as esophageal stenting, endoscopic clips, or endoscopic vacuum therapy.[9,43] In cases of large esophageal defects or poor tissue quality where repair or temporizing measure are felt to be unfeasible, esophagectomy to resect the affected patient may be considered.[44] In such cases, one can either restore continuity with a gastric or other conduit, or create a cervical esophagostomy. The selection of treatment modality for the esophageal injury depends on the clinical scenario, anatomic considerations, and overall patient stability, as well as available expertise and resources.

Esophageal-Atrial Fistulae

By contrast, when an EAF is present, several reports in the literature favor primary intracardiac repair on central cardiopulmonary bypass with an aortic cross clamp via a midline sternotomy, followed by either immediate or delayed esophageal repair.[42,45–47] This treatment sequence acknowledges that the largest cause of morbidity and mortality in this population is the entrainment of air or particulate matter from the esophagus into the vascular system, which can result in ischemic strokes and other systemic ischemic injuries. While the esophageal injury may be accessed through the posterior pericardium for repair via a midline sternotomy, the mid-esophageal location of these fistulae makes a right chest approach more favorable for exposure, particularly for perforations that extent beyond the field visible through sternotomy.[42] A thoracotomy incision also permits harvesting and use of an intercostal muscle flap to buttress the repair. Therefore, repositioning the patient, reintubating with double-lumen endotracheal tube to facilitate single-lung ventilation, and converting to a right posterolateral thoracotomy may be necessary.

During such an approach, one aims for minimal manipulation of the heart until the heart has been drained and the aortic cross-clamp has been placed to avoid air entry into the circulation or massive hemorrhage into the esophagus.[38] One must first place the patient on cardiopulmonary bypass; reports describe central aortic and bicaval venous canulation with a left ventricular vent to provide optimal decompression.[46] Once the aortic cross-clamp has been placed, the heart can be lifted to examine the posterior pericardium and identify the fistulous connection. The left atrium should be mobilized from the esophagus if possible. Use of a stapling device across the fistulous tract has also been described.[47] The atrial and esophageal defects should be directly inspected; flexible esophagoscopy can also be used for luminal visualization of the esophageal defect.

Primary intracardiac repair should be performed for the atrial defect. The atrial side of the fistula tract can be accessed via a left atriotomy in Sondergaard's groove. Once the fistula is identified via visual inspection or probing, the edges should be debrided to healthy tissue. Depending on the size of the defect, it can then be repaired either primarily with nonabsorbable monofilament suture, or with a pericardial patch.[44] Larger or more complex defects may require more creative reconstruction.[48]

Next, the esophageal defect should be identified and repaired. These are often repaired primarily in 2 layers using absorbable suture. A leak test may be performed with air or methylene blue. The repair should then be buttressed with healthy tissue, with could be an intercostal muscle flap, a pericardial flap, an omental flap, or others. Again, if the esophageal defect is too large or the tissue quality is inadequate for primary repair, resection and diversion should be considered.

Acknowledging the complexity and morbidity of this 2-stage surgical approach, some have advocated for a single-stage, on-pump or off-pump atrial and esophageal repair via a right posterolateral thoracotomy approach.[44,49,50] In such cases, if femoral cannulation for peripheral cardiopulmonary bypass was not established at the onset of the surgery, the groins should be left exposed for emergent cannulation if needed. Others have reported a single-stage approach where the fistula to the atrium was ligated without formal intracardiac repair.[51]

At the conclusion of the case, surgical drains should be placed to widely drain the pleural cavities, the mediastinum, and the pericardium. Consideration should also be given to the patient's ongoing nutritional need, and the placement of a gastrostomy or jejunostomy tube should be considered.

Patients should receive the appropriate postoperative care, including critical care management, as needed. At some point during the recovery, a contrast esophagogram can be performed to confirm an intact esophageal repair.

ALTERNATIVE INTERVENTIONAL MODALITIES

Esophageal stenting, which is often used for management of esophageal perforations, has also been described for the treatment of EAF and EPF.[14,52–55] Stenting has also been used as a temporizing measure prior to surgical intervention, or could be considered after failed surgical repair.[47] Other endoscopic techniques include endoscopic clipping. However, when an EAF is present, attempting endoscopy with air insufflation may allow air to pass into the systemic circulation, a scenario with potentially devastating consequences. Some have suggested a saline only endoscopy as an alternantive. Moreover, available data suggest worse outcomes for patients treated with endoscopic approaches compared to surgical repair.[2,53]

Patients treated nonsurgically must also have appropriate drainage, whether surgical or minimally invasive, of the pleural and pericardial spaces.

OUTCOMES

EAFs and EPFs are grim diagnoses, with significant morbidity and mortality. Although limited to the post-ablation population, the POTTER-AF study provides the most comprehensive data to date on outcomes following EAF.[2] The most common complications following presentation and treatments were sepsis or septic shock (57.9%), coma (46.7%), stroke or cerebral hemorrhage (23.4%), cardiac arrest (18.7%), gastrointestinal bleeding (16.8%), and cardiac tamponade (11.2%). Most patients were treated with surgical management with or without prior endoscopic intervention (47.4%), with 19.8% receiving endoscopic therapy alone and 32.8% receiving conservative management. Overall mortality was 65.8% (n = 77/117), with patients treated with operative (51.9%, n = 28/54) and endoscopic (56.5%, n = 13/23) interventions having a significantly lower mortality rate than those treated conservatively (89.5%, n = 34/38). The authors do acknowledge the significant selection bias that impacts the assessment of these treatment-based mortality rates, since the cohort treated with conservative management tended to have had a longer time to diagnosis and to be more critically ill.

SUMMARY

Fistulae between the esophagus and the pericardium or the left atrium are rare but feared complications of transcatheter ablations and esophageal procedures and pathologies. Patients may present variably with cardiopulmonary, gastrointestinal, and/or neurologic symptoms. A high index of suspicion is paramount to enable timely diagnosis, stabilization, and treatment. Our understanding of treatment strategies stems from case series and reports, with the presence of atrial involvement dictating the approach and extent of necessary interventions. Esophageal-pericardial fistulae may be approached via the right chest, with pericardial drainage and primary esophageal repair buttressed by a tissue flap. For esophageal-atrial fistulae, several reports favor primary intracardiac repair via median sternotomy on cardiopulmonary bypass with aortic cross-clamp, followed by esophageal repair. Endoscopic therapies may be used as primary or adjunctive treatment strategies for the esophageal injury. While mortality is high overall, surgical intervention confers the highest likelihood of survival.

CLINICS CARE POINTS

- Fistulae between the esophagus and the pericardium or the left atrium are rare but feared complications of transcatheter ablation procedures and esophageal procedures and pathologies.

- Patients may present variably with cardiopulmonary, gastrointestinal, and/or neurologic symptoms. A high index of suspicion is paramount to enable timely diagnosis and treatment.

- Multiple chest imaging modalities—including plain radiography, computed tomography, contrast esophagogram, echocardiogram, and esophagogastroduodenoscopy—may aid in establishing the diagnosis, with computed tomography being most used.

- Initial stabilization should include intravenous antimicrobial therapy; cardiopulmonary resuscitation, support, and emergent drainage; neurologic evaluation in cases of cerebral embolization; and nutritional support.

- Esophageal-pericardial fistulae may be repaired via a right chest approach, with drainage of the pericardial space and primary esophageal repair buttressed by a tissue flap.

- Esophageal-atrial fistulae generally require primary intracardiac repair via median sternotomy on central cardiopulmonary bypass with aortic cross-clamp, followed by immediate or delayed esophageal repair, although single-stage approaches via right chest posterolateral thoracotomy and using peripheral bypass have been described.

- Endoscopic therapies may be used as primary or adjunctive treatment strategies for the esophageal injury.

- While mortality is high overall, surgical intervention confers the highest likelihood of survival.

DISCLOSURE

The authors have no relevant conflicts of interest to disclose.

REFERENCES

1. Schecter WP, Hirshberg A, Chang DS, et al. Enteric fistulas: principles of management. J Am Coll Surg 2009;209(4):484–91.
2. Tilz RR, Schmidt V, Pürerfellner H, et al. A worldwide survey on incidence, management, and prognosis of oesophageal fistula formation following atrial fibrillation catheter ablation: the POTTER-AF study. Eur Heart J 2023;44(27):2458–69.
3. Lambert DR, Llaneza PP, Gaglani RD, et al. Esophageal-atrial fistula. J Clin Gastroenterol 1987;9(3):345–9.
4. Meltzer P, Elkayam U, Parsons K, et al. Esophageal-pericardial fistula presenting as pericarditis. Am Heart J 1983;105(1):148–50.
5. Denglos P, Nuytens F, Piessen G. Oesophageal-pericardial fistula: a rare complication of radiation-induced oesophagitis. Eur J Cardio Thorac Surg 2020;58(5):1097–9.
6. Achouh P, Pouly J, Azarine A, et al. Atrio-esophageal fistula complicating esophageal achalasia. Interact Cardiovasc Thorac Surg 2011;13(2):211–3.
7. Luthi F, Groebli Y, Newton A, et al. Cardiac and pericardial fistulae associated with esophageal or gastric neoplasms: a literature review. Int Surg 2003;88(4):188–93. Available at: https://www.ncbi.nlm.nih.gov/pubmed/14717523.
8. Kaufman J, Thongsuwan N, Stern E, et al. Esophageal-pericardial fistula with purulent pericarditis secondary to esophageal carcinoma presenting with tamponade. Ann Thorac Surg 2003;75(1):288–9.
9. Włodarczyk J, Olechnowicz H, Kocoń P. Esophago-pericardial fistula during the course of primary esophageal carcinoma. Ann Thorac Surg 2008;86(6):1967–9.

10. Ghunaim M, Someili A, Mawardi M. Candida Cardiac Tamponade Secondary to Oesophageal-Pericardial Fistula: A Rare Presentation of Oesophageal Squamous Cell Carcinoma. Eur J Case Rep Intern Med 2022;9(3):003200.

11. Xie H, Tu L, Li X, et al. More attention should be paid to atrial-esophageal fistula, and not all atrial-esophageal fistulas are iatrogenic. Ann Transl Med 2023;11(10):372.

12. Servais EL, Stiles BM, Spector JA, et al. Gastropericardial fistula: a late complication of esophageal reconstruction. Ann Thorac Surg 2012;93(5):1729–31.

13. Ruiz-Elizalde AR, Haley MJ, Fisher JC, et al. Gastric tube-pericardial fistula: a remote complication of esophageal replacement for long gap esophageal atresia. J Pediatr Surg 2009;44(7):1440–2.

14. Khader Y, Ghazaleh S, Nehme C, et al. Esophagopericardial Fistula After Esophagectomy. Cureus 2021;13(3):e13753.

15. Bowman AW, DiSantis DJ, Frey RT. Esophagopericardial Fistula Causing Pyopneumopericardium. Radiol Cardiothorac Imaging 2020;2(6):e200417.

16. Sánchez-Quintana D, Cabrera JA, Climent V, et al. Anatomic relations between the esophagus and left atrium and relevance for ablation of atrial fibrillation. Circulation 2005;112(10):1400–5.

17. Kapur S, Barbhaiya C, Deneke T, et al. Esophageal Injury and Atrioesophageal Fistula Caused by Ablation for Atrial Fibrillation. Circulation 2017;136(13):1247–55.

18. Assis FR, Shah R, Narasimhan B, et al. Esophageal injury associated with catheter ablation for atrial fibrillation: Determinants of risk and protective strategies. J Cardiovasc Electrophysiol 2020;31(6):1364–76.

19. Calkins H, Kuck KH, Cappato R, et al. 2012 HRS/EHRA/ECAS Expert Consensus Statement on Catheter and Surgical Ablation of Atrial Fibrillation: recommendations for patient selection, procedural techniques, patient management and follow-up, definitions, endpoints, and research trial design. Europace 2012;14(4):528–606.

20. Halbfass P, Pavlov B, Müller P, et al. Progression From Esophageal Thermal Asymptomatic Lesion to Perforation Complicating Atrial Fibrillation Ablation: A Single-Center Registry. Circ Arrhythm Electrophysiol 2017;10(8). https://doi.org/10.1161/CIRCEP.117.005233.

21. Nair GM, Nery PB, Redpath CJ, et al. Atrioesophageal fistula in the era of atrial fibrillation ablation: a review. Can J Cardiol 2014;30(4):388–95.

22. Ghia KK, Chugh A, Good E, et al. A nationwide survey on the prevalence of atrioesophageal fistula after left atrial radiofrequency catheter ablation. J Intervent Card Electrophysiol 2009;24(1):33–6.

23. Gandjbakhch E, Mandel F, Dagher Y, et al. Incidence, epidemiology, diagnosis and prognosis of atrio-oesophageal fistula following percutaneous catheter ablation: a French nationwide survey. Europace 2021;23(4):557–64.

24. Awadelkarim A, Shanah L, Ali M, et al. Esophago-Pericardial Fistulae as a Sequela of Boerhaave Syndrome and Esophageal Stenting: A Case Report and Review of Literature. J Investig Med High Impact Case Rep 2021;9. https://doi.org/10.1177/23247096211036540. 23247096211036540.

25. Park JK, Goto T, Nagano T, et al. Cerebral arterial air emboli after stent insertion in esophageal cancer complicated with esophago-left atrial fistula: An autopsy case and review of the literature. Pathol Int 2019;69(11):662–6.

26. Dagres N, Anastasiou-Nana M. Prevention of atrial-esophageal fistula after catheter ablation of atrial fibrillation. Curr Opin Cardiol 2011;26(1):1–5.

27. Sanchez J, Woods C, Zagrodzky J, et al. Atrioesophageal Fistula Rates Before and After Adoption of Active Esophageal Cooling During Atrial Fibrillation Ablation. JACC Clin Electrophysiol 2023;9(12):2558–70.

28. Dai WL, Yao KX, Li MM, et al. A novel esophageal retractor with eccentric balloon during atrial fibrillation ablation. Pacing Clin Electrophysiol 2023;46(9):1056–65.

29. Di Biase L, Saenz LC, Burkhardt DJ, et al. Esophageal capsule endoscopy after radiofrequency catheter ablation for atrial fibrillation: documented higher risk of luminal esophageal damage with general anesthesia as compared with conscious sedation. Circ Arrhythm Electrophysiol 2009;2(2):108–12.

30. Scanavacca M, Pisani C, Rivarola EWR. Early identification of oesophageal lesions after atrial fibrillation ablation to prevent atrio-oesophageal fistula. Eur Heart J 2023;44(47):5004–5.

31. Rivarola EWR, Moura E, Chou M, et al. A novel treatment for esophageal lesions following atrial fibrillation ablation. J Cardiovasc Electrophysiol 2021;32(3):713–6.

32. Grubina R, Cha YM, Bell MR, et al. Pneumopericardium following radiofrequency ablation for atrial fibrillation: insights into the natural history of atrial esophageal fistula formation. J Cardiovasc Electrophysiol 2010;21(9):1046–9.

33. French KF, Garcia C, Wold JJ, et al. Cerebral air emboli with atrial-esophageal fistula following atrial fibrillation ablation: a case report and review. Neurohospitalist 2011;1(3):128–32.

34. Giacomino BD, Worden N, Marchigiani R, et al. Pericardial-esophageal fistula complicating cryoballoon ablation for refractory atrial fibrillation. HeartRhythm Case Rep 2017;3(1):2–6.

35. Zakaria A, Hipp K, Battista N, et al. Fatal esophageal-pericardial fistula as a complication of radiofrequency catheter ablation. SAGE Open Med Case Rep 2019;7. https://doi.org/10.1177/2050313X19841150. 2050313X19841150.

36. Back Sternick E, Soares Correa F, Ferber Drumond L, et al. Esophago-pericardial fistula after catheter ablation of atrial fibrillation: A review. J Cardiovasc Electrophysiol 2020;31(10):2600–6.

37. Khan M, Rashid MU, Zafar H, et al. A Rare Complication of Cardiac Ablation: Atrial-esophageal Fistula Presenting as Odynophagia. Cureus 2020;12(2): e6871.

38. Sylvin EA, Jassar AS, Kucharczuk JC, et al. Pericardial-Esophageal Fistula: A Rare but Increasing Complication of Cardiac Ablation. Thorac Cardiovasc Surg Rep 2022;11(1):e27–9.

39. Khan MY, Siddiqui WJ, Iyer PS, et al. Left Atrial to Esophageal Fistula: A Case Report and Literature Review. Am J Case Rep 2016;17:814–8.

40. Wuestenberghs F, Pirson N, Bulpa P, et al. Iatrogenic cerebral air embolism revealing an atrial-esophageal fistula. Intern Emerg Med 2017;12(5):715–6.

41. Osuna Garibay AS, Arroyo-Rodríguez C, Victoria-Nandayapa JR, et al. Tension pneumopericardium secondary to esophageal-pericardial fistula. Rev Port Cardiol 2022;14. https://doi.org/10.1016/j.repc. 2021.09.021.

42. Tauber K, Singhal S, Jarrar D, et al. Optimal Surgical Approach to Left Atrioesophageal Fistula After Catheter Radiofrequency Ablation. Ann Thorac Surg 2022;114(3):e161–3.

43. Watkins JR, Farivar AS. Endoluminal Therapies for Esophageal Perforations and Leaks. Thorac Surg Clin 2018;28(4):541–54.

44. Dulac AS, Lebreton G, Vaillant JC, et al. Atrio-esophageal fistula: Surgical management. J Visc Surg 2023;160(5):368–73.

45. Gray WH, McFadden PM. Commentary: In left atrial esophageal fistula repair there is more than one way to "skin the cat": Just remember "first things first.". JTCVS Tech 2020;4:173–4.

46. Gray WH, Fleischman F, Cunningham MJ, et al. Optimal Approach for Repair of Left Atrial-Esophageal Fistula Complicating Radiofrequency Ablation. Ann Thorac Surg 2018;105(5):e229–31.

47. Guenthart BA, Sun B, De Biasi A, et al. Surgical technique for atrial-esophageal fistula repair after catheter ablation: An underrecognized complication. JTCVS Tech 2020;4:169–72.

48. Chen LW, Chen JY, Fang GH, et al. Novel Approach for Repair of a Left Atrial Esophageal Fistula After Radiofrequency Ablation. Ann Thorac Surg 2021; 111(3):e205–7.

49. Shimamura J, Moussa F, Tarola C, et al. Surgical Repair of Atrial-Esophageal Fistula Following Catheter Ablation. Ann Thorac Surg 2022;113(4):e275–8.

50. Duda A, Beers K, Mitiek M. Surgical management of atrial-esophageal fistula as a complication of atrial fibrillation ablation. J Surg Case Rep 2022;2022(1): rjab497.

51. Lee J, Yoon J, Hong SB, et al. One-step thoracotomy approach for atrial-esophageal fistula repair without cardiopulmonary bypass. Gen Thorac Cardiovasc Surg 2023;71(11):681–4.

52. Fairbairn K, Worrell SG. Esophageal Perforation: Is Surgery Still Necessary? Thorac Surg Clin 2023; 33(2):117–23.

53. Zhou B, Cen XJ, Qian LY, et al. Treatment strategy for treating atrial-esophageal fistula: esophageal stenting or surgical repair?: A case report and literature review. Medicine 2016;95(43):e5134.

54. Verma V, Bhyan P, Patel JM, et al. Esophageal-Pericardial Fistula: A Rare Complication of Atrial Fibrillation Catheter Ablation Treated Successfully With an Esophageal Stent: 606. Journal of the American College of Gastroenterology | ACG 2015;110:S268. Available at: https://journals.lww.com/ajg/fulltext/ 2015/10001/esophageal_pericardial_fistula__a_rare. 606.aspx. [Accessed 4 January 2024].

55. Ormanci D, Doğanay K, Ari H, et al. The way to a patient's heart is through their esophagus: A case of esophago-pericardial fistula. Echocardiography 2022;39(12):1627–30.

Airway Esophageal Fistula

Kelsey E. Koch, MD, Andrew P. Dhanasopon, MD, Gavitt A. Woodard, MD*

KEYWORDS

- Tracheoesophageal fistula • Acquired airway fistula • Malignant fistula • Surgical TEF repair
- Esophageal stenting • Airway stenting

KEY POINTS

- Acquired trachea esophageal fistulas (TEFs) can occur due to various causes such as trauma, infection, mechanical ventilation, iatrogenic injuries, surgical complications, consequences of radiation treatment, and malignancy.
- Evaluation and management of a suspected TEF requires accurate localization of the fistulous connection, and treatment in the context of the etiology, patient comorbidities, and nutrition status.
- Definitive surgical repair is the optimal treatment for long-term control of ongoing contamination and return to oral nutrition, but stenting has become a viable option in select cases.
- For surgical repair of proximal TEFs, a transverse cervical incision is performed, with proximal or distal extension if needed along the lateral neck or sternum, respectively. For distal TEFs, especially when located near the carina, surgical repair should be approached through a right thoracotomy. Repair strategies include isolation and division of the fistulous tract, and primary closure of the defects with local muscle flap for separation and buttressing.
- Esophageal and airway stents for TEFs can be utilized in select cases such as a bridge to definitive surgical repair, or symptom management in malignant TEFs.

INTRODUCTION

Acquired tracheoesophageal fistulas (TEFs) are rare pathologic connections between the trachea and esophagus that are life-threatening due to ongoing contamination of the lower respiratory system and malnutrition with prolonged illness. Common causes of acquired TEFs include esophageal malignancy, prior radiation treatment, complications from surgery including esophagectomy, trauma, iatrogenic injuries, infection, and inflammatory reactions such as erosion due to foreign bodies including excessively inflated balloon cuffs from endotracheal/tracheostomy tubes. Approximately half of TEFs arise from cancers of the esophagus, lung, larynx, trachea, thyroid, or involved lymph nodes.[1,2] Esophageal carcinoma is reported to be the most common cause of malignant TEFs due to the proximity of the esophagus and trachea.[1] The diagnostic challenge in either benign or malignant etiologies is distinguishing from aspiration; symptoms often include recurrent cough or pneumonia despite multiple courses of medical treatment, and persistent dysphagia. Prompt evaluation and treatment are the keys to preventing and reducing ongoing contamination of the lower respiratory system. Treatment will depend on the location and etiology of the TEF and patient factors such as comorbidities and nutritional status, and all of which are critical to optimal outcomes. This article focuses on the evaluation and management of patients with acquired TEFs.

EVALUATION

Diagnosis of acquired TEFs tends to be delayed due to the rarity of the diagnosis and symptom overlap with other more common conditions. On average, patients with TEFs due to malignancy are diagnosed approximately 7 months after symptom onset. Acquired TEFs can lead to a variety of symptoms depending on etiology, size, location,

Division of Thoracic Surgery, Yale School of Medicine, 330 Cedar Street, BB205, New Haven, CT 06520, USA
* Corresponding author.
E-mail address: gavitt.woodard@yale.edu

Thorac Surg Clin 34 (2024) 405–414
https://doi.org/10.1016/j.thorsurg.2024.07.005
1547-4127/24/© 2024 Elsevier Inc. All rights are reserved, including those for text and data mining, AI training, and similar technologies.

and patient nutritional status. Most common symptoms include coughing after swallowing (known as "Ono's sign"), worsened with carbonated drinks, dysphagia, aspiration, fever, pneumonia, hemoptysis, shortness of breath, and chest pain.[3–5]

In ventilated patients, symptoms like unexplained weight loss, recurrent chest infections, difficulty weaning off ventilation, increased secretions during suctioning, and pneumonia due to tracheal soiling should raise concern for development of a TEF. Positive pressure ventilation through the fistula can lead to gastric dilation with continued, unexplained air-leak from the ventilator circuit.[5–7]

DIAGNOSTIC STUDIES

There are no formal guidelines for the diagnosis and treatment of acquired TEF. Contrast esophagram has historically been the initial diagnostic test of choice, although its sensitivity varies depending on type of contrast given, swallowing status of the patient, and the experience of the radiologic technician and radiologist performing the test who utilize various positions and maneuvers to visualize the suspected location. Orally or endoscopically administered contrast that shows communication with the trachea or bronchial tree is diagnostic for TEF (**Fig. 1**). Barium has been used as the standard contrast due to its superior mucosal coating and radiographic density compared to water-soluble Gastrograffin. Gastrograffin also carries the well-known risk of pneumonitis if aspirated, which is of particular concern when a TEF is suspected.[8–10] Contrast

esophagram has been shown to accurately identify the TEF in approximately 70% of patients.[11,12] Computed tomography (CT) with intravenous contrast and oral barium contrast enhancement is also commonly used to confirm TEF if oral contrast is detected within the airways (assuming normal swallowing function). In the authors' practice, a contrast esophagram, immediately followed by CT scan with intravenous contrast, provides the confirmation of TEF by 2 different imaging modalities and anatomic information including presence of lung parenchymal and/or pleural space infection.

While imaging is the most expedient, least invasive diagnostic test, the most sensitive method is esophagoscopy. When located in the distal bronchial tree, sensitivity may be as high as 97%.[1,13] Depending on the potential need for surgery and on the practice environment, it can be advantageous for the surgeon to perform the diagnostic endoscopy for localization and preoperative planning. Whether by surgeon or gastroenterologist, diagnosis relies on careful mucosal examination, visualization despite often limited ability to insufflate due to the TEF, and if needed, confirmation of TEF with contrast injection and subsequent bronchoscopic clearance of contrast.[6] (**Fig. 2**) Bronchoscopy is commonly used in conjunction with esophagoscopy to confirm the TEF location and increase the diagnostic yield. By itself, bronchoscopic visualization is only successful in about 46% of cases. However, similar to esophagoscopy, a complete bronchoscopic evaluation of the airway by the surgeon provides valuable information for operative planning.[14]

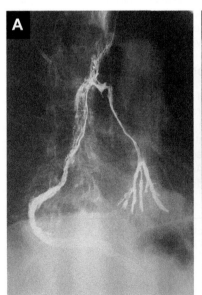 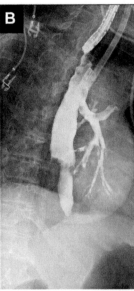

Fig. 1. (*A*, *B*) Barium administration during upper endoscopy demonstrating communication of esophageal contrast with bronchial tree.

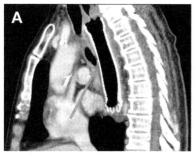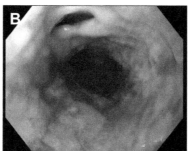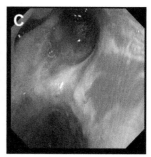

Fig. 2. (*A*) Chest computed tomography (CT) scan of a patient with an esophageal stent in place for benign stricture following radiation treatment of non-small cell lung cancer. With the esophageal stent in place, a tracheaelesophageal fistula (TEF) developed and is evident on CT with loss of tissue planes between the membranous airway and stent (*orange arrow*). (*B*) Upper endoscopy of the same patient following stent removal shows fistula site within the esophageal lumen. (*C*) Flexible bronchoscopy performed during the same procedure shows site of the fistula in the left main stem bronchus membranous airway.

MANAGEMENT

Once a diagnosis and determination of etiology have been made, effective management requires evaluation of patient comorbidities, nutritional status, and discussion of goals of therapy. Strategies to minimizing airway contamination by the esophagus include stopping oral intake, gastric acid-reducing medications (such as proton pump inhibitors and H2-receptor antagonists), and especially for intubated patients, care management such as elevating the head of bed and frequent oral suctioning. For mechanically ventilated patients, endotracheal tube advancement with cuff insufflation distal to the identified TEF should be performed to prevent contamination of the airway due to retrograde reflux of any esophageal contents. For TEFs involving the distal airways, a bronchial blocker in the affected side may prevent contamination of the contralateral respiratory tract. Orogastric or nasogastric tubes may be placed to further reduce the risk of gastric reflux, but care should be taken to ensure side ports are not located near the TEF, to avoid any negative pressure necrosis that may worsen the TEF. If a gastrostomy tube will be placed for nutrition access, consideration could be made for gastro-jejunal tube that would allow gastric drainage and concurrent jejunal feeding.

OPERATIVE MANAGEMENT

Surgery is the most definitive treatment option. The goal of surgical treatment is primary closure of the TEF and prevention of recurrence with intervening viable tissue flap achieved in a single-stage repair. The decision between the approaches depends on the specific characteristics of the case, the surgeon's expertise, and the patient's condition, with a consideration for potential benefits and drawbacks associated with each method.[15,16]

ANTERIOR CERVICAL APPROACH

For proximal, cervical TEFs, a transverse cervical incision has been described, with sternal extension if needed for additional exposure. Compared to a lateral cervical approach, the anterior, transverse cervical incision provides a wider, more direct access to the trachea. This increased exposure is best utilized when managing larger fistulas and especially when associated with tracheal stenosis. The patient should be positioned on the table with a shoulder bump and the neck extended. Early communication with the anesthesia team is critical, ensuring they are prepared to perform cross-table ventilation. Bronchoscopy-assisted intubation is performed to ensure both appropriate placement of the cuff distal to the fistula and to ensure the tube does not intubate the esophagus through the defect. A transverse incision approximately 10 cm is made 2 fingerbreadths above the sternal notch. Soft tissue is divided, ensuring strap muscle is preserved for later flap, and the thyroid divided. The pretracheal fascia is opened in a longitudinal fashion and dissection may be carried as inferiorly as the level of the carina if needed for mobilization. Bronchoscopy is utilized to identify the location of the fistula so circumferential dissection of the trachea can be performed at the correct level, minimizing the risk of devascularization or recurrent laryngeal nerve injury.

Dependent upon the size of the fistula, either primary repair or complete resection can be completed. If the fistula measures less than 5 mm, repair can be approached by creating an anterior tracheotomy and sharply dividing the fistulous tissue directly, debriding any inflammatory tissue in a transtracheal fashion. Once the fistula is divided, the trachea can be retracted, and the esophageal defect repaired in 2 layers with an inner absorbable suture and an outer non-absorbable suture. The esophageal repair is tested for leaks with endoscopy and insufflation. A pedicled strap muscle flap is then secured over the esophageal repair. The posterior tracheal defect is reapproximated with absorbable suture and the anterior tracheotomy closed with absorbable suture.[17,18]

If the fistula measures greater than 10 mm or tracheal stenosis is present, the trachea can be transected and the distal airway intubated on table allowing ventilation while the remaining repair can be performed. The portion of trachea transected should be kept less than 4 cm to ensure a tension-free anastomosis. The TEF is carefully separated from the esophagus and opened along its length. The esophageal mucosa is reapproximated with absorbable suture and the muscular layer reapproximated with permanent suture. The esophageal repair is tested for leaks with endoscopy and insufflation. A pedicled strap muscle flap is then positioned over the esophageal repair and the tracheal ends anastomosed with absorbable suture.[17,18] The trachea is reconstructed end to end with absorbable suture, passing the endotracheal tube distally and resuming ventilation once the posterior membrane is reapproximated. The surgical field is filled with warm saline, the endotracheal tube cuff is deflated, and positive pressure leak test applied to test the anastomosis.

This method follows the principle of segmental tracheal resection and anastomosis with primary esophageal closure followed by buttressing the repair with pedicled muscle flap. The muscle flap is a critical step to place viable tissue between the esophageal repair and the tracheal-tracheal anastomosis to prevent recurrent fistula formation. Benefits of this approach include excellent exposure of the fistula, decreased risk to the recurrent laryngeal nerve, and a low incidence of tracheal stenosis as the abnormal segments are entirely removed and the anastomoses are not aligned, minimizing the risk of recurrent fistula.[19] It is a complex but well-structured procedure with multiple safeguards to ensure a successful repair while minimizing complications.

LEFT LATERAL CERVICOTOMY

For cervical and cervicothoracic junction fistulae, a left lateral cervicotomy has been described. The patient is positioned with their head tilted to the right; an incision is made along the anterior border of the left sternocleidomastoid. If needed, the incision may be extended through a partial sternotomy for increased exposure, especially if access to the mediastinum is necessary. The platysma is divided and the sternocleidomastoid, carotid sheath, and descending hypoglossal nerve are identified and retracted laterally. The thyroid and larynx are retracted medially, allowing for identification and preservation of the recurrent laryngeal nerve. With endoscopic guidance, transillumination can be used to identify the level of the fistula and the esophagus can be bluntly dissected circumferentially. It is often helpful to have a naso/orogastric tube to help palpate and identify the esophagus. The TEF can then be divided and the edges of the trachea and esophagus debrided. The esophagus is closed in 2 layers and the trachea repaired with an absorbable suture and the closure confirmed with leak tests as described earlier. This approach allows exposure of the entire esophagus from the cricoid to the superior mediastinum, providing exposure of the fistulous tract.[20] An interposition muscle flap can be placed between the 2 repairs, or the esophagus can be rotated to separate the repairs and fixed to the prevertebral plane.[18]

Compared to an anterior, transverse cervical approach, the left lateral cervicotomy exposure is more limited, more likely to cause tissue devascularization due to more mobilization, and increased risk of recurrent laryngeal nerve injury, although the left-sided approach aims to minimize nerve injury, given the more predictable course of the recurrent laryngeal nerve as compared to the right. It is best utilized in the setting of small fistulas, measuring less than 5 mm, without associated tracheal stenosis.[6]

RIGHT THORACOTOMY

A right thoracotomy is reserved for distal TEFs, located at or near the tracheal carina. The patient is intubated with either a double-lumen endotracheal tube, or a single-lumen endotracheal tube and the left mainstem bronchus intubated. Upper endoscopy and flexible bronchoscopy are performed for confirmation of the anatomy, location of the TEF opening within the esophagus and airway, and bronchoscopic clearing of secretions. If an esophageal stent is in place, this can be initially left in place as an anatomic guide to be removed later during the case. When no esophageal stent is in place, anasogastric or orogastric tube (NGT) can be placed at this time as an anatomic guide to identify the esophagus. After being positioned in left lateral decubitus, a right posterolateral thoracotomy is performed in the fourth intercostal space. The distal trachea and both main bronchi are secured to aid in the dissection and exposure. The esophagus is mobilized to allow for elevation and rotation. Similar to the methods described earlier, the fistula is identified by either bronchoscopy or endoscopy and the esophagus is carefully separated from the trachea to expose the entire fistula. Once completely exposed, the fistula is divided and the esophagus and tracheal tissues debrided. As described earlier, the esophageal and tracheal ends are reapproximated. The repairs examined and tested with endoscopy and insufflation in the esophagus and hyperinflation with a deflated cuff to evaluate the tracheal repair.[21] In rare instances of large TEF, prior extensive radiation or inflammation, esophagectomy with esophago-gastric anastomosis may be considered but care must be taken to place muscle flap between the conduit anastomosis and the repaired membranous airway. In instances of a large membranous airway defects, several repairs approaches are possible. The membranous airway can be patched with bovine pericardium with muscle flap for buttressing (**Fig. 3**). Direct muscle flap coverage of the defect in the membranous airway has also been described.

STENTING

Stenting as a method to exclude the TEF on the esophageal and/or tracheal side has been typically performed as a bridge to definitive surgical repair, especially for benign etiologies, or for palliative reasons when major surgery is not advisable or not within the patient's goals of care, especially in cases of advanced malignancy.[22–25] For either situation, the size of the lumen being stented and the device's radial force exerted need to be taken into consideration. An oversized stent may lead to enlargement of this fistula and decreased mucosal perfusion[6,25,26] The decision regarding the type of esophageal and/or tracheal stent, quantity, and location of stents are critical and require careful consideration by clinicians. There are a variety of stents available, including self-expanding metallic stents, silicone stents, covered or uncovered

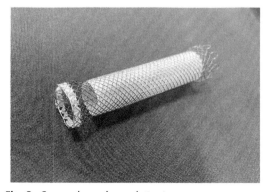

Fig. 3. Covered esophageal stent.

stents, and biodegradable stents (**Table 1**). Each type has its advantages and limitations in terms of durability, flexibility, ease of placement, and potential complications. The choice often depends on the specific characteristics of the fistula and the patient's condition. Determining the number of stents needed involves assessing the size and extent of the fistula. In some cases, a single stent might suffice, while larger or more complex fistulas might require multiple stents to adequately seal the abnormal connection. Additionally, the precise placement of the stent is crucial as it needs to cover the entire length of the fistula to provide an effective seal. Factors like the proximity to the carina, the esophagus's diameter, and the position of the fistula in relation to anatomic structures influence where the stent should be positioned.[25,27]

ESOPHAGEAL STENTING

Esophageal stents are effective in in the mid to distal portions of the esophagus, especially in patients without known airway stenosis. In benign TEFs, stenting often serves as a temporary measure before definitive surgery.[26] In contrast, stenting is considered a more definitive treatment in patients with malignant TEF.[27,28] Self-expandable plastic stents are commonly used due to their ease of retrieval, minimizing the impact the stent would have on the planned surgical repair. Only 1 self-expanding plastic stent, the Polyflex stent, has Food and Drug Administration (FDA) approval for use in benign esophageal disease.[29] Self-expandable metallic stents (SEMSs) are often preferred due to their durability, effectiveness in managing a wide range of malignant esophageal diseases, and resistance to tumor ingrowth. Covered SEMSs resist tumor ingrowth better but have a higher risk of migration compared to uncovered SEMSs while partially covered SEMSs have the benefit of decreased migration risk; however, this comes with increased difficulty in stent removal.[30] (**Fig. 4**) Partially uncovered SEMSs may shorten on expansion, and therefore, care must be taken in stent selection to account for the shortening.[31] Current commercially available stent options are listed in **Table 1**. All patients should undergo an esophagram following stent placement to confirm no leakage of contrast around the proximal and distal landing zones of the stent placement before resuming feeding. If leakage persists, oversizing or additional proximal/distal stenting may seal these endoleaks.[31]

Complications from esophageal stenting can include extrinsic airway compression, bleeding, esophageal perforation, and the formation of new fistulas. Paradoxically, stent placement might

Table 1
Esophageal stents

Stent	Covered/Uncovered	Manufacturer	Material
Polyflex	Covered	Boston Scientific	Polyester (silicone coating)
Ultraflex (covered)	Covered	Boston Scientific	Nitinol (polyurethane coating)
Ultraflex (noncovered)	Uncovered	Boston Scientific	Nitinol
WallFlex Partially Covered	Partially covered	Boston Scientific	Nitinol (silicone coating)
WallFlex Fully Covered	Covered	Boston Scientific	Nitinol (silicone coating)
Z-Stent with Dua Anti-Reflux Valve	Covered	Cook Medical	Stainless steel (polyurethane coating)
Evolution Fully Covered	Covered	Cook Medical	Nitinol (internal and external silicone coating)
Evolution Partially Covered	Partially covered	Cook Medical	Nitinol (internal and external silicone coating)
Bonastent	Covered	EndoChoice	Nitinol (silicone coating)
Alimaxx-ES	Covered	Merit Medical Endotek	Nitinol (polyurethane coating)
Alimaxx-E	Covered	Merit Medical Endotek	Nitinol (polyurethane coating, inner silicone coating)
Niti-S Double Stent	Covered	Taewoong Medical Co	Nitinol (polyurethane outer coating)
Niti-S Covered Stent (fully covered)	Covered	Taewoong Medical Co	Nitinol (polyurethane inner and outer coating)

sometimes lead to the development of new TEFs.[30,32] In cases where there is an elevated risk of airway obstruction due to extrinsic compression by the esophageal stent, simultaneous stenting of both the airway and esophagus (double stenting) might be considered in selected circumstances.

TRACHEAL STENTING

The 2 primary materials used for airway stents are silicone and metal. In malignant TEFs, self-expandable metallic stents are preferred as they are easier to deploy, achieve good apposition to the airway mucosa, potentially minimize migration, and provide strong radial expansile forces. They can also be placed with either flexible or rigid bronchoscopy and do not require fluoroscopy, making placement easier in technically challenging locations. They also offer ease of revision immediately after deployment. The metal is less durable when compared to silicone, which contributes to higher rates of stent fracture; however, durability is less

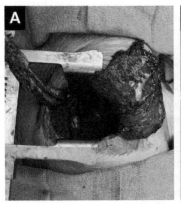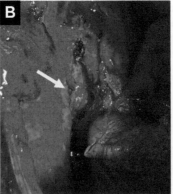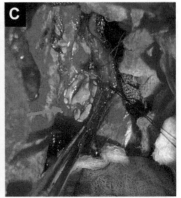

Fig. 4. (*A*) Operative repair of TEF via a right thoracotomy with mobilization of latissimus and intercostal muscle flaps. (*B*) In this case, given prior extensive damage to the esophagus and poor-quality tissues, an esophagectomy was planned. Here, the esophagus has been opened and the fistulous connection to the bronchus can be seen (*yellow arrow*). (*C*) Bovine pericardial patch repair of the membranous airway was performed (*blue arrow*) and covered in muscle flaps. Esophagectomy was then performed with a neck anastomosis.

concerning in malignant TEF as these patients rarely outlive the stent.[33] Comparatively, silicone stents are available in Y-shaped configurations for fistulas at the carina and have external studs to reduce mucosal ischemia and prevent migration; however, these studs can make repositioning more challenging and may hinder complete apposition to the airway wall, posing challenges in obtaining a seal overlying the TEF.[34,35] In terms of durability, silicone stents are more durable compared to metal stents, making them potentially more favorable in managing benign TEFs.[33] Current commercially available bronchial and tracheal stents are listed in **Table 2**.

The location of the fistula may contribute to the decision to stent the trachea instead of the esophagus, with proximal TEFs unfavorable for esophageal stent. Ideally, the deployed stent should cover the entire fistula with a 20 mm landing zone proximally and distally. Achieving this margin may be challenging depending on the fistula's location.[25]

DOUBLE STENTING

The use of double stenting or simultaneous placement of stents in the esophagus and trachea as a primary intervention in managing TEFs is a debated practice. However, it can be considered, particularly in cases where there is a perceived risk of airway compromise despite proper sizing and deployment of the esophageal stent. Double stenting is intended to serve as a protective measure against airway compression by esophageal stents and to prevent

migration into the airway.[23,26] The airway stent is placed first followed by esophageal stents to mitigate airway compromise risks. The proximal end of the esophageal stent is placed higher than the upper margin of the airway stent to reduce esophageal stent migration. Unfortunately, friction or pressure necrosis between the luminal surfaces of the airway and esophageal stents, especially with metal-on-metal contact, can pose a risk of fistula enlargement which is the primary reason this practice is reserved for unique circumstances.[21,25,36]

While these strategies are adopted based on anecdotal successes and smaller case series, the efficacy and comparative outcomes of single versus double stenting remain a topic of contention. Clinicians often employ these strategies based on individual patient factors, experience, and the perceived risk of complications to mitigate the challenges associated with TEF management.

NOVEL ENDOSCOPIC TECHNIQUES

In addition to stenting, there are several other endoscopic closure techniques to address TEFs in poor surgical candidates. Many of the treatment options can be used simultaneously and many are reported to have greater success when used in combination. Overall, the morbidity and mortality of endoscopic closure are lower than surgical repair, as is the successful closure rate. Size and chronicity are both factors in the likelihood of successful closure of TEFs.[37]

Table 2				
Tracheal and bronchial airway stents				
Stent	**Mechanics**	**Material**	**Advantages**	**Disadvantages**
Bonastent	Self-expanding	Nitinol (silicone coating)	Compatible with flexibility bronchoscopy	Migration, fracture
Silmet	Self-expanding	Nitinol (silicone coating)	Customizable	Migration, fracture
Hanarostent	Self-expanding	Nitinol (silicone coating)	Compatible with flexibility bronchoscopy	Migration, fracture
Carina-Y-Stent	Self-expanding	Nitinol (elastic coating)	Multiple shapes with various coating	Migration, fracture
COMVI	Self-expanding	Nitinol (polytetrafloroethylene coating)	Triple layered	Migration, fracture
iCAST	Balloon expandable	Stainless steel (polytetrafloroethylene coating)	Low profile	Migration
Dynamic	Rigid stent	Stainless steel (silicone coating)	Resists collapse	Laryngoscopy required

Over-the-scope clips (OTSC) have high rates of full-thickness closure and are relatively easy to use; however, their utility is limited to small-diameter TEFs. Successful closure of TEF using OTSC is reported up to 90%; however, long-term efficacy rates are poor.[38] Endoscopic suturing is another method that ensures adequate approximation of tissues. Unfortunately, this technique has poor long-term closure rates and requires skill and familiarity with endoscopic suturing techniques.[37]

Tissue sealants, like fibrin glue, thrombin, and cyanoacrylate, have also been used and demonstrate efficacy, most notably when used with other methods and on very small (<5 mm) fistulas. Most data for tissue sealants are found in the pediatric population. The risks of sealants include leaking of sealant into the airway causing potential plugging.[39] In addition to occlusion, sealants work through different mechanisms including inflammation and tissue necrosis. Like sealant, argon plasma coagulation and polyglycolic acid sheets are technically easy to apply and are most likely to be successful when combined with other methods.

Cardiac septal occlusion devices have also been reported with relatively high initial reported efficacy, although limited data. Complications include TEF enlargement and airway obstruction. Vacuum-assist devices have also been reported with successful closure rates of 85%. This method requires frequent endoscopic evaluation and sponge exchange and requires transnasal suction tubing for at least 3 weeks.[37]

OUTCOMES

Although still rare, the management of TEFs has improved over the last few decades with high rates of successful management and good quality of life in benign disease with reported curative rates of 93% to 96% in patients managed with surgical repair.[19,20,37,40] Recurrence rates for benign fistulas were lower with surgical repair compared to stent placement, with reported rates of 21% and 63%, respectively.[37,41]

Malignant or post esophagectomy fistulas have a lower rate of success, with institutions reporting successful surgical closure rates of 50% to 60%.[37,42,43] Unfortunately, malignant TEFs are associated with a much higher mortality rate, with median overall survival of 36 months post diagnosis and a reported 5-year survival of only 21%.[42,43] In patients with malignant TEF who undergo stent placement as management, technical success rates are reported at 100%; however, patient outcomes remain poor as this is a palliative treatment strategy and mortality is driven by the underlying malignancy.[37]

SUMMARY

Tracheoesophageal fistulas encompass a wide spectrum of causes, symptoms, diagnostic methods, and various treatment modalities. A prompt and accurate diagnosis using imaging techniques such as contrast esophagography, CT scans, and endoscopic procedures is imperative. Early identification and subsequent management are crucial, especially considering the varied symptoms and potential life-threatening complications associated with TEFs. The principles of treatment for TEF are to prevent ongoing soilage of the airway for infection control and provide options for long-term enteral nutrition. Approaches for surgical management depend on location and patient factors. Successful repair requires fistula division and closure of the defect on both esophageal and airway side, interposition of a pedicled muscle flap, and optimization of patient comorbidities. Stenting remains an option for both a bridging technique in benign TEF and a palliative treatment in malignant TEF if successful seal over the leak can be achieved. The different stent options as well as the associated risks and benefits must be considered when choosing the most suitable stent type, size, and placement based on the individual characteristics of the fistula and the patient's condition. Double stenting remains a debated but potential intervention in specific cases, emphasizing the need for a careful balance between managing airway compromise and potential complications associated with the stents. Advances in diagnostic testing, treatments, and critical care continue to improve outcomes in patients with TEF.

CLINICS CARE POINTS

- Definitive surgical repair remains the optimal management of tracheal esophageal fistulas but stenting can be considered as a temporizing measure or in patients who are not surgical candidates.

- Principles of surgical management are isolation and division of the fistulous tract and primary closure with or without tracheal or esophageal resection with local muscle flap interposition for separation and buttressing.

- Despite prompt diagnosis and optimal care, tracheal esophageal fistulas are a life threatening problem and are often diagnosed in patients with pulmonary infections and poor nutritional status. Attempts should be made to medically optimize patients if possible prior to surgical resection.

DISCLOSURE

G. Woodard reports participation in advisory boards for AstraZeneca. G. Woodard reports research funding support from Thoracic Surgery Foundation, International Association for the Study of Lung Cancer Young Investigator Award, and Yale SPORE in Lung Cancer (P50 CA196530). Others have nothing to disclose.

REFERENCES

1. Reed MF, Mathisen DJ. "Tracheoesophageal fistula". Chest Surg Clin N Am 2003;13(2):271–89.
2. Davydov M, Stilidi I, Bokhyan V, et al. "Surgical treatment of esophageal carcinoma complicated by fistulas". Eur J Cardio Thorac Surg 2001;20(2):405–8.
3. Burt M, Diehl W, Martini N, et al. "Malignant esophagorespiratory fistula: management options and survival". Ann Thorac Surg 1991;52(6):1222–9.
4. Gerzić Z, Rakić S, Randjelović T. "Acquired benign esophagorespiratory fistula: report of 16 consecutive cases". Ann Thorac Surg 1990;50(5):724–7.
5. Diddee R, Shaw IH. "Acquired tracheo-oesophageal fistula in adults". Cont Educ Anaesth Crit Care Pain 2006;6(3):105–8.
6. Khemasuwan D, Griffin D. "Management of acquired tracheoesophageal fistula in adults". In: Turner Jr, Francis J, Jain P, et al, editors. From thoracic surgery to interventional pulmonology: a clinical guide. Cham: Springer International Publishing; 2021. p. 117–33.
7. Kim HS, Khemasuwan D, Diaz-Mendoza J, et al. "Management of tracheo-oesophageal fistula in adults". Eur Respir Rev 2020;29(158):1–11.
8. Bohl JL, Timmcke AE. "Radiology". In: Beck DE, Roberts PL, Saclarides TJ, et al, editors. The ASCRS textbook of colon and rectal surgery. New York, NY: Springer New York; 2011. p. 77–106.
9. Gore RM, Levine MS. Textbook of gastrointestinal radiology. 4th edition. Philadelphia: Elsevier/Saunders; 2015.
10. James AE, Montali RJ, Chaffee V, et al. "Barium or gastrografin: which contrast media for diagnosis of esophageal tears? ". Gastroenterology 1975;68(5). https://doi.org/10.1016/S0016-5085(75)80222-8.
11. Little BP, Mendoza DP, Fox A, et al. "Direct and indirect CT imaging features of esophago-airway fistula in adults". J Thorac Dis 2020;12(6):3157.
12. Couraud L, Ballester MJ, Delaisement C. "Acquired tracheoesophageal fistula and its management". Semin Thorac Cardiovasc Surg 1996;8(4).
13. Zhou C, Hu Y, Xiao Y, et al. "Current treatment of tracheoesophageal fistula". Ther Adv Respir Dis 2017; 11(4):173–80. SAGE Publications Ltd.
14. Mammana M, Pangoni A, Lorenzoni G, et al. "Adult benign, non-iatrogenic bronchoesophageal fistulae: systematic review and descriptive analysis of individual patient data". World J Surg 2021;45(11): 3449–57.
15. Thomas AN. "The diagnosis and treatment of tracheoesophageal fistula caused by cuffed tracheal tubes". J Thorac Cardiovasc Surg 1973;65(4). https://doi.org/10.1016/s0022-5223(19)40744-7.
16. Bartlett RH. "A procedure for management of acquired tracheoesophageal fistula in ventilator patients". J Thorac Cardiovasc Surg 1976;71(1). https://doi.org/10.1016/s0022-5223(19)40264-x.
17. Grillo HC. Surgery of the trachea and bronchi. USA: PMPH; 2004.
18. Shen KR, Allen MS, Cassivi SD, et al. "Surgical management of acquired nonmalignant tracheoesophageal and bronchoesophageal fistulae". Ann Thorac Surg 2010;90(3):914–9.
19. Kim SP, Lee J, Lee SK, et al. "Surgical treatment outcomes of acquired benign tracheoesophageal fistula: a literature review". J Chest Surg 2021;54(3). https://doi.org/10.5090/jcs.21.012.
20. Marulli G, Loizzi M, Cardillo G, et al. "Early and late outcome after surgical treatment of acquired nonmalignant tracheo-oesophageal fistulae". Eur J Cardio Thorac Surg 2013;43(6). https://doi.org/10.1093/ejcts/ezt069.
21. Santosham R. "Management of acquired benign tracheoesophageal fistulae". Thorac Surg Clin 2018; 28(3):385–92.
22. Blackmon SH, Santora R, Schwarz P, et al. "Utility of removable esophageal covered self-expanding metal stents for leak and fistula management". Ann Thorac Surg 2010;89(3). https://doi.org/10.1016/j.athoracsur.2009.10.061.
23. Colt HG, Meric B, Dumon JF. "Double stents for carcinoma of the esophagus invading the tracheobronchial tree". Gastrointest Endosc 1992;38(4):485–9.
24. Dumonceau JM, Cremer M, Lalmand B, et al. "Esophageal fistula sealing: choice of stent, practical management, and cost". Gastrointest Endosc 1999;49(1):70–8.
25. Hürtgen M, Herber SCA. "Treatment of malignant tracheoesophageal fistula". Thorac Surg Clin 2014; 24(1):117–27.
26. Freitag L, Tekolf E, Steveling H, et al. "Management of malignant esophagotracheal fistulas with airway stenting and double stenting". Chest 1996;110(5). https://doi.org/10.1378/chest.110.5.1155.
27. Herth FJF, Peter S, Baty F, et al. "Combined airway and oesophageal stenting in malignant airway-oesophageal fistulas: a prospective study". Eur Respir J 2010;36(6). https://doi.org/10.1183/09031936.00049809.
28. Sreedharan A, Harris K, Crellin A, et al. "Interventions for dysphagia in oesophageal cancer". Cochrane Database Syst Rev 2009;4. https://doi.org/10.1002/14651858.CD005048.pub2.

29. Hindy P, Hong J, Lam-Tsai Y, et al. "A comprehensive review of esophageal stents". Gastroenterol Hepatol 2012;8(8).

30. Izumi A, Yoshio T, Sasaki T, et al. "Efficacy and safety of self-expandable metallic stent placement for malignant esophageal fistula". J Clin Med 2023;12(18). https://doi.org/10.3390/jcm12185859.

31. Adler D. Self-expanding stents in gastroenterology, . Thorofare. United States: SLACK Incorporated; 2012 [Online]. Available at: http://ebookcentral.proquest.com/lib/yale-ebooks/detail.action?docID=3404588. Accessed April 9, 2024.

32. Eroglu A, Turkyilmaz A, Subasi M, et al. "The use of self-expandable metallic stents for palliative treatment of inoperable esophageal cancer". Dis Esophagus 2010;23(1). https://doi.org/10.1111/j.1442-2050.2009.00978.x.

33. Chang CH, Lin J. "Management of aero-digestive fistulas in adults: the bronchoscopist's perspective". Mediastinum 2023;7. https://doi.org/10.21037/MED-22-38/COIF.

34. Wang H, Tao M, Zhang N, et al. "Airway covered metallic stent based on different fistula location and size in malignant tracheoesophageal fistula". Am J Med Sci 2015;350(5). https://doi.org/10.1097/MAJ.0000000000000565.

35. Avasarala SK, Freitag L, Mehta AC. "Metallic endobronchial stents: a contemporary resurrection". Chest 2019;155(6). https://doi.org/10.1016/j.chest.2018.12.001.

36. Shamji FM, Inculet R. "Management of malignant tracheoesophageal fistula". Thorac Surg Clin 2018; 28(3):393–402.

37. Nehme F, Ge PS, Coronel E. "Management of aero-digestive fistulas: the gastroenterologist's perspective, a narrative review". Mediastinum 2023;7. https://doi.org/10.21037/MED-22-48/COIF.

38. Haito-Chavez Y, Law JK, Kratt T, et al. "International multicenter experience with an over-the-scope clipping device for endoscopic management of GI defects (with video)". Gastrointest Endosc 2014; 80(4):610–22.

39. Meier JD, Sulman CG, Almond PS, et al. "Endoscopic management of recurrent congenital tracheoesophageal fistula: a review of techniques and results". Int J Pediatr Otorhinolaryngol 2007;71(5): 691–7.

40. Koch M, Vasconcelos Craveiro A, Mantsopoulos K, et al. "Analysis of surgical treatment strategy and outcome factors in persistent tracheoesophageal fistula: a critical analysis of own cases and review of the literature". Eur Rev Med Pharmacol Sci 2022;26(1). https://doi.org/10.26355/eurrev_202201_27776.

41. Aworanti O, Awadalla S. "Management of recurrent tracheoesophageal fistulas: a systematic review". Eur J Pediatr Surg 2014;24(5). https://doi.org/10.1055/s-0034-1370780.

42. Zheng B, Zeng T, Yang H, et al. "The clinical characteristics, treatments and prognosis of post-esophagectomy airway fistula: a multicenter cohort study". Transl Lung Cancer Res 2022;11(3). https://doi.org/10.21037/tlcr-22-141.

43. Bertrand T, Mercier O, Leymarie N, et al. "Surgical cervicothoracic-flap repair of neoesophagus–airway fistula after esophagectomy for esophageal cancer: a retrospective cohort study". JTCVS Tech 2024. https://doi.org/10.1016/j.xjtc.2023.10.027.

Conduit Ischemia After Esophagectomy
A Spectrum of Clinical Manifestations, Prevention, and Management

Megan Turner, MD*, Nicholas Baker, MD

KEYWORDS

- Esophagectomy • Gastric conduit necrosis • Gastric conduit ischemia • Anastomotic leak

KEY POINTS

- Esophagectomy remains a cornerstone in the standard of care for esophageal cancer, in addition to a solution to other end-stage esophageal pathologies and a bailout for widely contaminated esophageal perforations. Despite this, it is often associated with significant morbidity, particularly regarding complications associated with conduit ishcemia.
- The gastric conduit relies on the right gastroepiploic for blood supply, with an extensive network of submucosal capillaries solely responsible for the perfusion of the proximal conduit and, thus, the esophageal anastomosis. As such, the proximal conduit and anastomosis are prone to ischemic complications, which exist on a spectrum ranging from submucosal ischemia to leak to conduit necrosis.
- Ischemic complications affect both short- and long-term patient outcomes. Many have proposed mechanisms to avoid ischemic complications, whether by preoperative conduit conditioning, intraoperative techniques to assess conduit perfusion, management of perioperative hypotension, and prevention of conduit distension. The most commonly used methods are discussed here.
- With ischemic complications do occur, early identification and treatment are paramount. Both clinical and laboratory parameters (e.g. white blood cells, C-reactive protein) are used to raise suspicion, with esophagram, computed tomography (CT), or esophagogastroduodenoscopy use to confirm the diagnosis. Historically, esophagram has been the gold standard for confirming leaks. However, CT scans are increasingly favored with or without oral contrast.
- With ischemic complications do occur, early identification and treatment are paramount. Both clinical and laboratory parameters (e.g. white blood cells, C-reactive protein) are used to raise suspicion, with esophagram, computed tomography (CT), or esophagogastroduodenoscopy use to confirm the diagnosis. Historically, esophagram has been the gold standard for confirming leaks. However, CT scans are increasingly favored with or without oral contrast.
- As ischemic complications manifest on a spectrum so too does their management– starting with conservative approaches with antibiotics +/- drain placement, progressing to endoscopic interventions, often with stent placement, and beyond to surgical interventions with conduit revision or conduit takedown with bipolar exclusion depending on the extent of conduit ischemia and mediastinal contamination.

Department of Cardiothoracic Surgery, University of Pittsburgh Medical Center, 200 Lothrop Street, Pittsburgh, PA 15213, USA
* Corresponding author.
E-mail address: turnerm11@upmc.edu

Thorac Surg Clin 34 (2024) 415–425
https://doi.org/10.1016/j.thorsurg.2024.05.004
1547-4127/24/© 2024 Elsevier Inc. All rights are reserved, including those for text and data mining, AI training, and similar technologies.

CONDUIT ISCHEMIA–LEAK AND NECROSIS
Introduction

Esophagectomy remains a gold standard for successfully treating early-stage and locally-advanced esophageal cancers in combination with neoadjuvant chemoradiation. Esophagectomy is also a viable surgical treatment for end-stage achalasia in patients who have failed myotomy, severely symptomatic and refractory esophageal dysmotility disorders, or in cases of esophageal or foregut perforation and sepsis. Despite refinements in surgical technique, including the advent of minimally invasive laparoscopic and robotic approaches since its conception in 1913, the complication rate and associated morbidity of esophagectomy remains as high as 66% at 30 days.[1] Of all potential complications, however, none is as feared as conduit ischemia. The manifestations of this complication comprise a spectrum, ranging from a focal area of mucosal ischemia detected incidentally to an anastomotic leak or, at its extreme, complete conduit necrosis. Conduit ischemia thus encompasses a wide range of pathology and presentations—on which both anastomotic leak and conduit necrosis sit—driven by impaired blood supply to or from some part and thickness of the conduit, resulting in tissue death and breakdown.

Anastomotic leak following esophagectomy is commonly quoted to occur at a rate of about 11.4%. It is more common in cervical anastomosis (12%) than in intrathoracic anastomosis (9%) for reasons further discussed later in this article.[2] In 2015, the Esophagectomy Complications Consensus Group (ECCG) formally defined anastomotic leak as "a full-thickness gastrointestinal defect involving the esophagus, anastomosis, staple line, or conduit irrespective of presentation or method of identification," classifying leaks as being type I-III (**Table 1**) depending on the degree of intervention, if any, required to treat.[3] Conduit necrosis, or death of part or all of the conduits, is reported in most series with an incidence of 1 to 3%—presumably accounting for only instances of extensive necrosis rather than submucosal ischemia or focal ischemia resulting in leak.[4–9] In most esophagectomies, the stomach is the conduit used to replace the esophagus, although the jejunum and colon are also options. The ECCG also set grading for gastric conduit necrosis, again ranging from type I-III (**Table 2**), based on the invasiveness of required treatment.[3] Understanding the physiologic and anatomic basis for gastric conduit ischemia, technical and patient-related risk factors, prevention methods, strategies for early detection, and management options for the

Table 1
Classification of anastomotic leak by Esophagectomy Complications Consensus Group

Type of Leak	Definition
Type I	Local defect requiring no change in therapy or treated medically or with dietary modification
Type II	Localized defect requiring interventional but not surgical therapy (eg, drain placement, stent, bedside I&D)
Type III	Localized defect requiring surgical therapy

From Low, D.E., Alderson, D., Cecconello, I., Chang, A.C., Darling, G.E., D'Journo, X.B., Griffin, S.M., Hölscher, A.H., Hofstetter, W.L., Jobe, B.A., Kitagawa, Y., Kucharczuk, J.C., Law, S.Y.K., Lerut, T.E., Maynard, N., Pera, M., Pera, M., Peters, J.H., Pramesh, C.S., Reynolds, J.V., Smithers, B.M., van Lanschot, J.J.B. International Consensus on Standardization of Data Collection for Complications Associated With Esophagectomy: Esophagectomy Complications Consensus Group (ECCG). Ann Surg. 2015; 262(2):286-294.

Table 2
Classification of conduit necrosis by Esophagectomy Complications Consensus Group

Type of Necrosis	Definition/ Characteristics	Treatment Required
Type I	Conduit necrosis focal—identified endoscopically, superficial	Managed with additional monitoring or non-surgical therapy
Type II	Conduit necrosis focal—identified endoscopically, not associated with free anastomotic or conduit leak	Surgical therapy does not involve esophageal diversion.
Type III	Conduit necrosis extensive	Conduit resection with diversion

From Low, D.E., Alderson, D., Cecconello, I., Chang, A.C., Darling, G.E., D'Journo, X.B., Griffin, S.M., Hölscher, A.H., Hofstetter, W.L., Jobe, B.A., Kitagawa, Y., Kucharczuk, J.C., Law, S.Y.K., Lerut, T.E., Maynard, N., Pera, M., Pera, M., Peters, J.H., Pramesh, C.S., Reynolds, J.V., Smithers, B.M., van Lanschot, J.J.B. International Consensus on Standardization of Data Collection for Complications Associated With Esophagectomy: Esophagectomy Complications Consensus Group (ECCG). Ann Surg. 2015; 262(2):286-294.

resulting complications is of utmost importance to the thoracic surgeon, as anastomotic leak has been associated with an increase in 30-day mortality, decreased quality of life, and increased cancer recurrence rates—while frank mediastinal sepsis from extensive conduit necrosis can reach a mortality rate of 90%.[2,4,6,7,10] This article aims to explore these tenets and further discuss the impact of these complications in patients who survive them.

Anatomy of the Conduit

As stated earlier, the most used conduit for esophagectomy is the stomach, which will be discussed in the most details in this article. The blood supply to the stomach and the steps required to mobilize it during an esophagectomy appropriately leaves the proximal portion of the stomach or conduit—and therefore the anastomosis—inherently at risk of ischemia.

The stomach is supplied on its lesser curve by the left and right gastric arteries, on its greater curve by the left and right gastroepiploics, and on its fundus by the short gastrics. From each of these vessels, a dense submucosal capillary network is formed. During esophagectomy, the stomach is extensively mobilized and fashioned into a tube along the greater curvature, leaving the conduit dependent upon the right gastroepiploic arcade alone for its blood supply. However, this vessel typically extends to only 60% of the length of the conduit, leaving the perfusion of the proximal end of the conduit (ie, the fundus) dependent on the aforementioned capillary network.[2,5] It is typically in this region of the conduit in which the anastomosis is fashioned, particularly in cervical anastomosis, which requires a longer conduit length. The necessary narrowing of the stomach as it is tubularized stands to disrupt the submucosal network upon which the proximal conduit and anastomosis are reliant for blood supply. While narrower conduits expedite emptying, many theorize that narrowing beyond the established 4 cm may compromise to the submucosal network. However, this has not been explored in randomized control trials (RCTs) for widths less than 4 cm.[2] With an already tenuous blood supply to the proximal conduit and anastomosis, great care must be taken to avoid further compromise to perfusion.

Risk Factors for Ischemia–Patient, Technique, Intra- and Post-op Management

As with most surgical complications, there are patient-specific factors that can predispose an individual to developing ischemia and anastomotic leak. Multiple studies have cited cardiac disease, coronary disease, peripheral arterial disease or stenosis of the celiac trunk, chronic kidney disease, diabetes, hypertension, malnutrition, obesity, steroid use, and tobacco use as contributing to the development of ischemia and leak.[4,7,8,11,12] Interestingly, neoadjuvant chemoradiation has not been associated with increased leak rate.[4,7,13] One must also consider prior abdominal surgeries and inflammatory pathologies, particularly those near the origin of the right gastroepiploic that may complicate dissection, that is, cholecystectomy, pancreatitis, and so forth.[14]

There are several technical points to consider when creating the conduit and anastomosis that may contribute to development of ischemia. The width of the conduit is considered to be a factor, as stated previously, with most surgeons preferring a conduit width of greater than or equal to 4 cm to avoid potential disruption of the submucosal capillary network.[2] One should also avoid twisting the conduit and maintaining the staple line parallel to the blood supply, as rotation can lead to compression, undue tension, and conduit distension. The conduit should remain decompressed postoperatively to prevent strain on the anastomosis and potential venous congestion. This is often accomplished temporarily by nasogastric tube insertion in the postoperative period. Many advocate for pyloroplasty, pyloromyotomy, or pyloric Botox to encourage conduit emptying, although there is controversy as to whether or not this indeed decreases leak rate.[10] Tension on the conduit and anastomosis should also be avoided, with complete mobilization of the stomach accomplished intraoperatively so that the pylorus can be pulled up to the hiatus without tension. The hiatus should also not be too tight to impair perfusion or emptying but not loose enough to allow for herniation, which can cause the same issues.[4,14]

Regarding the creation of the anastomosis itself, the key is mucosal apposition. Beyond this, no evidence supports increased rates of local ischemia or breakdown with stapled versus hand-sewn technique.[7,9,15,16] It should be noted, however, that when creating a stapled anastomosis, the gastrotomy used to introduce the stapler should be at least 2 to 3 cm separated from the actual anastomosis to avoid ischemia of the intervening tissue.[17] Studies have also been performed looking at the leak rate of an end-to-end versus end-to-side anastomosis, with the latter observed to have a significantly higher incidence of leak.[13,18] Many advocate buttressing the anastomosis with a vascularized omental pedicle, both to serve as a mechanical barrier to prevent gross contamination from small leaks but also, in theory, to encourage angiogenesis, given the high vascular endothelial growth factor expression within vascularized omentum, augmented in the setting of hypoxia.[19] A meta-analysis by Chen and colleagues in 2014 looking at 3 RCTs did reveal a significant reduction in leak with the addition of omentoplasty, both in cervical and intrathoracic anastomoses.[20] However, another meta-analysis, which included the same 3 trials when sub-stratifying patients based on the type of esophagectomy, found that this significant difference was only upheld in the transhiatal esophagectomy group.[21] Of note, patients undergoing neoadjuvant chemoradiation were excluded from the trials used for this meta-analysis. Lu and colleagues published a single-center, multi-surgeon retrospective study on omentoplasty in patients who had undergone neoadjuvant treatment and did not find a significant difference in either leak rate or the need for leak-related operation. It should be noted, however, that this study included far fewer patients and was retrospective.[19] Finally, it is well-established that cervical anastomoses have a higher leak rate in comparison to intrathoracic anastomoses—12.3% versus 9.3%— theorized to be in part due to increased risk of tension, increased compression at the thoracic inlet, and the necessity of a longer gastric conduit, placing the anastomosis in a region of the conduit with a more tenuous blood supply.[7,11,16]

It should also be noted that there is no evidence to support increased rates of ischemia and subsequent leak or necrosis in open versus minimally invasive esophagectomy (MIE), either laparoscopic or robot-assisted. However, a definite learning curve exists for transitioning to a minimally invasive technique.[4,14–10,22]

Finally, hypotension represents the most significant risk factor for ischemia both in the intra- and post-operative period, again due to the tenuous blood supply to the distal conduit. Many advocate avoiding vasopressors, given the small-caliber vessels supplying the tip of the conduit, instead favoring volume. However, this must also be measured against the risk of venous congestion. There have been multiple studies looking at the relationship between vasopressor use and anastomotic leak without demonstration of a relationship. A recent retrospective study by Walsh and colleagues (2021) did not reveal an increased leak rate in patients who received intraoperative pressor with conservative fluid administration, aiming to maintain systolic blood pressure greater than 90 mm Hg. Furthermore, in those that did develop a leak, there was no link between the severity of the leak and pressor use.[23] It should be noted, however, that no explicit algorithm was used to direct volume or pressor administration. In the same vein, epidural analgesia has often been used as an adjunct in pain management for esophagectomy patients and often results in hypotension from systemic absorption of the analgesics. Multiple studies demonstrated that countering this with intraoperative phenylephrine could reverse any resulting malperfusion without increased risk of leak.[7] While there undoubtedly needs to be a balance between fluid administration and conservative pressor use, the adequate treatment and prevention of hypotension is the most critical factor to avoid compromising conduit perfusion.

Novel Techniques for Prevention of Ischemia and Ischemic Complications

Apart from the operative technique itself, surgeons have sought both pre- and intra-operative interventions to minimize the risk of ischemia. Several studies have examined the effect of ischemic preconditioning in the pre-operative setting. This technique, first proposed by Urschel and colleagues in 1997, involves surgical ligation or angioembolization of all or some of the vessels to the stomach divided during esophagectomy to allow neo-angiogenesis to occur before conduit formation. Studies have suggested 4 to 5 days for the microcirculation and perfusion of the stomach to return to baseline following esophagectomy, with subsequent neovascularization of the submucosa reaching a peak around 14 days.[24–28] Thus, most proponents of the procedure suggest at least 14 days between ischemic preconditioning and esophagectomy. The data on whether there is an actual decrease in incidence of ischemia and leak following ischemic preconditioning is mixed, and often heterogeneous regarding method (laparoscopic vs angioembolic), and the specific vessels ligated. An RCT by Mils and colleagues in 2022 involving 28 patients undergoing Ivor-Lewis esophagectomy showed a significant reduction in ischemia-related events in the group assigned to angioembolism ischemic preconditioning. However, this may have been bolstered by the relatively high leak rate in the control group, quoted at 33%.[27] A meta-analysis in 2023 by Aiolfi and colleagues, which included both laparoscopic and angioembolism methods, as well as single- and multivessel techniques, also showed a reduction in the cumulative incidence of leak in patients who underwent preconditioning (8.8% vs 14.4%) with a respiratory rate (RR) of 0.63 (CI 0.47–0.86), as well as a reduction in the incidence of conduit necrosis (0.2% vs 1.9%). However, the RR was not significant.[24] There have also been reports of decreased severity—assessed by intervention required—of leak following ischemic preconditioning.[24,28] However, one must also consider the added risk of complications with these procedures. In regards to the laparoscopic technique, this adds an additional invasive surgical procedure and risk of surgical complications and allows the formation of additional adhesions that may complicate later esophagectomy. The angioembolism method is less invasive but can result in dissection of vessels, splenic infarction or necrosis, necrotizing cholecystitis, pancreatitis, and access site bleeding.[24] In the study mentioned earlier by Mils and colleagues, 22.7% of those who underwent the angioembolism preconditioning experienced complications—most frequently dissection of target vessels.[27] With these considerations, the risk-to-benefit ratio may only favor the procedure in patients at higher risk for ischemia-related complications.[24]

In the intraoperative setting, the focus has been on identifying gastric tip ischemia prior to creating the anastomosis to allow resection of any poorly perfused areas of conduit. Intraoperative doppler has been used to confirm the integrity of the right gastroepiploic along the length of the conduit; however, it may be less reliable in the proximal portion of the conduit relying on a submucosal network. Various methods have been proposed to augment gross visual assessment, but perhaps the simplest and most readily available is fluorescence imaging with indocyanine green (ICG). This involves the intravenous (IV) administration of ICG and the use of a specialized camera to detect the dye, with the intensity of the uptake of the dye in the tissue corresponding to the degree of perfusion.[7] A single-center, single-surgeon study involving 40 patients performed by Dalton and colleagues in 2017, which designated 20 patients to undergo an intraoperative assessment with ICG, failed to find a significant difference between the ICG and non-ICG group in the incidence of the leak. Six of the 20 patients in the experimental group underwent additional conduit resection based on ICG data– 2 of these still had postoperative leak.[29] More extensive testing will be needed to determine the utility of this intervention in the future.

DIAGNOSIS OF ANASTOMOTIC LEAK, CONDUIT ISCHEMIA

The development of leak or conduit necrosis usually occurs within the first 2 weeks postoperatively or even within the first 1 to 3 days postoperatively should there be a technical issue.[7] As discussed previously, the morbidity of ischemia-related complications, whether it be leak or conduit necrosis, is significant, contributing to increased mortality, decreased quality of life, and increased rates of disease recurrence in the setting of malignancy.[7,10] As such, early detection and treatment of these complications is critical. Despite this, the most appropriate use of adjuncts to the clinical examination—whether specific laboratory tests, imaging, or endoscopy—is widely debated. This section will outline the typical clinical findings, laboratory tests, imaging, and procedural adjuncts used to detect ischemic complications.

Clinical presentation may range from subtle to overt sepsis and shock depending on the degree of mediastinal contamination—with the latter typically seen in cases of extensive gastric conduit necrosis. Patients may exhibit any combination of fevers, tachycardia, new-onset atrial fibrillation, respiratory distress, delirium, or even bad breath secondary to bacterial overgrowth within necrotic tissue. Most surgeons elect to leave a drain near the anastomosis to assess for any leak visually and hopefully allow for complete control of small leaks. The appearance of a leak within a drain may be bilious or even frothy. One may also note an accumulation of air in a gravity drainage bag or, in the case of a Jackson-Pratt bulb, failure to hold suction. In some cases, the drain may not capture the leak effluent, and these characteristics can be seen in the pleural drain.

Laboratory tests can serve as an early indication of ischemic complications even before overt clinical manifestations. A persistent or increasing leukocytosis is concerning; however, it may be underwhelming in a well-drained leak. Many advocate for using C Reactive Protein (CRP) trends postoperatively, with a persistent elevation or rise in CRP beyond postoperative day (POD) 3 as indicative of possible leak.[7,30] It seems the trend of CRP is most useful beyond POD 3, as an exact cutoff value is challenging to establish. However, most studies agree a value at or greater than 170 mg/L on POD 3 is significant, with higher numbers achieving greater sensitivity. Specifically, a reported sensitivity of 176 mg/L on POD 3 was reported to have a sensitivity of 74%, with a value of 190 mg/L having a sensitivity of 100%.[1,7] Still, neither leukocytosis nor CRP are specific for these complications. Drain amylase level has been used as an adjunct to detect leaks, either following a change in drain character or as a routine assessment, usually on postoperative days 3 to 4. Again, no set cutoff value has been established, with some studies citing values as low as 31 IU/L and as high as 250 IU/L for a POD 4 cutoff, with sensitivities ranging from 75% to 100% and specificities ranging from 52% to 95.5%.[1,7] In reality, a combination of clinical picture and laboratory studies should be utilized to raise suspicion, with confirmation of diagnosis typically occurring through imaging and endoscopic adjuncts.

The main radiographic methods for assessing the conduit and anastomosis are the esophagram and computed tomog‐graogy (CT) chest, often with oral contrast. Practices vary depending on the institution, whether a routine imaging study is obtained at a set post-operative interval in the absence of other signs or ordered solely when a complication is suspected. Those who perform routine imaging generally do so to direct the resumption of oral intake. However, critics argue a normal result on 1 day does not preclude the development of a leak or necrosis at a later date and clinical suspicion will ultimately direct further investigation in these cases.[7] Imaging remains a critical diagnostic tool for anastomotic leak and conduit necrosis.

Historically, esophagrams have been the gold standard for diagnosing leaks, typically with water-soluble contrast followed by barium if the swallow is negative but suspicion remains high. However, while the test's specificity has been reported to approach 100% in some studies, the sensitivity of diagnosis is rather abysmal, ranging from 33% to 52%, with inferior results for cervical anastomoses.[1,7] In addition, there is the inherent risk of aspiration on contrast administration, with possible aspiration pneumonia or pneumonitis. CT chest, usually with IV contrast, has thus emerged as a diagnostic alternative, often with the administration of positive oral (PO) contrast just before imaging to allow assessment of extraluminal contrast. CT has the benefit of not just identifying leaks but potentially identifying partial-thickness conduit necrosis in cases with no extravasation of contrast, undrained mediastinal collections, or ongoing pneumonia. Again, the risks associated with PO contrast use are not eliminated, and the sensitivity and specificity are variably improved depending on the study, contrast adjuncts, and radiologist interpretation, with some studies reporting sensitivities closer to 55% and others touting values closer to 85%. Specificity is generally captured in the 80s to 90s % range, increased with PO contrast.[1,4,7] One of the frequent confounders in the interpretation of CT for this purpose is the presence of mediastinal air and to what degree it can be considered "normal" in the postoperative setting. One study by Shoji and colleagues in 2018 attempted to develop a guideline for interpretation of the quantity of mediastinal air on CT as indicative of a leak, dubbed the "air bubble sign," using patients who had undergone MIE with either cervical (majority) or intrathoracic anastomosis. The group performed non-contrast CT chest without the addition of PO contrast on POD 6 and interpreted a positive air bubble sign as 3 air bubbles in the mediastinum, with an air bubble itself defined as an air density larger than 2 mm in the minor axis and did not include those in contact with bone, drains, or surgical staples as these more likely represented artifact. Using this sign to identify a leak, sensitivity was reported at 86.4% and specificity at 95.8%. An esophagram was also performed on POD 7. Of the 22 patients diagnosed with a leak, 11 were not identified by esophagram, but 10 out of 11 did have a positive air bubble sign.[31] This technique had the added benefit of avoiding the risks of contrast aspiration. Whether these data can be reliably replicated, remains to be seen.

In nearly all leak and conduit necrosis cases, the diagnosis is confirmed using endoscopy. Visualization of the conduit and anastomosis is considered the gold standard, with sensitivity and specificity of 95%, allowing the identification of pinhole leaks and partial thickness necrosis that may otherwise be missed on imaging.[4,7] Endoscopy may be performed either in the operating room or bedside in the intensive care unit on intubated patients. The main drawbacks to endoscopy as a routine method for screening for ischemic complications is the time and resources required, the invasiveness of the procedure, and the fear of disrupting a fresh anastomosis. However, it has been documented that routine esophagogastroduodendroscopy within the first-week postop to assess anastomosis integrity and conduit viability can be done safely and that the intraluminal pressure from insufflation required for visualization does not itself pose a risk to anastomotic integrity.[6,7] In smaller leaks, endoscopy may serve as a diagnostic and therapeutic intervention, as detailed in the next section. Still, endoscopy does not provide a view of the extraluminal environment, and in cases of ischemic complications, obtaining a CT would still be advisable to assess for undrained collections. Given this, many advocate for CT imaging as first-line to either screen for or on suspicion of ischemic complications, with endoscopy to confirm diagnosis.[7]

In summation, it is a combination of clinical picture, laboratory values, and imaging studies that ultimately direct the surgeon to suspicion of leak or necrosis, and lead to confirmation of the diagnosis most often via endoscopy. The utility of screening asymptomatic patients during the first postoperative week, either via imaging or endoscopy, is debated. Still, the emphasis should remain on careful interpretation of the clinical and laboratory data to allow for early diagnosis and prompt management.

MANAGEMENT OPTIONS

Management of ischemic complications varies widely depending on the severity, from conservative measures in a small, contained leak or mucosal ischemia to resection of conduit and bipolar exclusion in cases of complete conduit necrosis. The tenants; however, remain the same—drainage, containment, and antibiotic coverage.

No surgical therapy is required for grade I anastomotic leak or conduit necrosis as set forth by the ECCG. For anastomotic leaks, this typically applies to tiny, pinhole leaks without undrained mediastinal collections, usually entirely controlled by a nearby anastomotic drain. For conduit necrosis, this typically applies to a focal partial-thickness or mucosal necrosis. In either case, these complications are typically managed by administering broad-spectrum IV antibiotics or antifungals, nutrition supplementation via jejunostomy tube, and an "nothing by mouth" or minimal clear liquid diet. Most surgeons also include antiacid agents (usually proton pump inhibitors), and some advocate for using anticholinergics to minimize saliva production and prokinetic agents to encourage conduit emptying. Patients often undergo serial endoscopies to monitor for resolution.[3,7] These noninvasive measures are additionally applied to the management of higher grades of leak and necrosis, as discussed I.

Grade II anastomotic leaks tend to involve a larger circumference of the anastomosis, leading to leakage of intraluminal contrast not entirely controlled by a perianastomotic drain. These necessitate additional intervention, either image-guided or endoscopic, but not surgical. In cervical anastomoses, often the cervical incision can be opened, irrigated, and packed to control the leak, provided there has not been contamination of the thoracic cavity. In thoracic anastomoses, additional localized collections not controlled by pleural or perianastomotic drains can be further managed by the placement of interventional radiology-guided drains. To avoid further contamination of the mediastinum, endoscopic therapies may be employed to seal the leak, including self-expandable metallic stents (SEMS), endoscopic vacuum therapy (EVAC), endoscopic clipping, or sealant.[7] SEMS are the most popular of these, followed by EVAC therapy. In general, SEMS should be used for leaks involving less than 70% of the anastomotic circumference, with some suggesting

avoiding their use in greater than 30% circumferential disruption.[7] Stents are generally left in place for 4 to 6 weeks to prevent tissue ingrowth. The average time for a leak to heal in conjunction with stent placement is 4 to 8 weeks, with efficacy cited at or more than 90% when used in the appropriate population and in conjunction with adequate drainage.[7,32,33] EVAC therapy can be utilized for more significant leaks—with reported use in even circumferential anastomotic breakdown—or those associated with a large abscess cavity. Setup involves the introduction of a polyurethane sponge either in the abscess cavity itself (intracavitary) or within the esophagogastric lumen at the site of dehiscence (intraluminal), which is then attached to a wound vac via a nasogastric tube. Healing via this method usually requires 12 to 36 days, with endoscopically-guided vac changes 1 to 2 times a week, making them more maintenance-intensive than SEMS. Success rates of this method are quoted at 86% to 100%.[7] Neither SEMS nor EVAC therapies are particularly successful in cervical anastomoses. Grade II conduit necrosis again describes a focal process, still without leakage of intraluminal contents. Still, unlike type I typically requires surgical intervention, given increased depth or surface area of affected tissue. Typically, this involves resectioning part of the conduit and recreating the anastomosis within a viable area of the conduit. Often, a vascularized, pedicled flap is used to reinforce the anastomosis, consisting of pedicled intercostal muscle, pleura, or pericardium for intrathoracic anastomoses, and sternocleidomastoid or pectoralis major for cervical anastomoses.[7]

Grade III anastomotic leaks tend to be more extensive, with diffuse contamination of the mediastinal or pleural space requiring surgical therapy for adequate drainage in addition to one of the endoscopic therapies discussed earlier, or in conjunction with resection of part of the conduit and refashioning of the anastomosis similar to management of grade II gastric necrosis. Grade III conduit necrosis is perhaps the most feared esophagectomy complication, describing diffuse necrosis of the conduit leading to uncontrolled leakage of intraluminal contents, mediastinitis, and sepsis. These patients are often critically ill and require prompt return to the operating room for resection of the dead conduit and bipolar exclusion—i.e., creation of an esophagostomy with reduction of any remaining gastric conduit to the abdomen, and placement of a G tube for drainage and a J tube for enteral nutrition. The maximal length of the remaining esophagus should be preserved at the initial exclusion to facilitate future reconstruction. Should the patient be too unstable to tolerate a more prolonged operation, resection of the dead tissue, irrigation, and drainage is the priority—the exclusion can be finalized after the patient is appropriately resuscitated. As mentioned previously, mortality of type III conduit necrosis approaches 90%. For those that do survive, the focus is on nutritional optimization and rehabilitation to restore gastrointestinal continuity. This can be done with a substernal pull-up of the remaining stomach in the rare instance that enough length is preserved, or more frequently with interposition of the jejunum or colon, also in the substernal position, with a cervical anastomosis performed in all cases.[1,6,7] To allow space for the new conduit to pass under the sternum and through the thoracic inlet without compression, the left hemi-manubrium and head of the left clavicle are resected, with some advocating for resection of the first rib as well. In jejunal interpositions, the jejunal conduit is typically "supercharged" via anastomosis of the second jejunal branch to cervical vessels—most frequently the left internal mammary—with the remainder of the blood supply coming from the vascular pedicle containing the fourth jejunal branch still connected to the native superior mesenteric artery. The leak rate for these esophagojejunal anastomoses is reported to be near 32%, with a 4% to 5% rate of graft necrosis and 10% combined in-hospital and 90-day mortality.[4,34] Colonic interpositions may be performed using the right or left colon. However, most surgeons prefer the left, given the smaller diameter and less variation in its blood supply, which is kept on a pedicle during interposition. The leak rate of esophagocolonic anastomosis is reported at 16% (specifically for cervical anastomoses), with graft necrosis around 5%.[4,6,34] Unlike jejunal grafts, colonic grafts are prone to dilation and subsequent redundancy, causing symptoms of dysphagia as the conduit fails to empty.[6,34] Alternative conduit options have been described for short-segment cervical conduit necrosis, including the use of muscle flaps—typically the sternocleidomastoid, pectoralis major, or trapezius—to partially reconstruct the conduit and cover the area of defect. Even rarer are short-segment fasciocutaneous free flaps utilizing a tubularized graft of skin from the forearm or thigh, although the failure rates for these are high.[4]

In cases of acute intraoperative conduit necrosis, options for rescue vary depending on stage of the operation and conduit used. An effort should first be made to eliminate any sources of impingement, including loosening of the hiatus or, in the case of a cervical anastomosis, increasing space in the thoracic inlet via further mobilization or

dissection, division of the interclavicular ligament, or in extreme cases, resection of a portion of the clavicle, manubrium, or rib.[4,5] However, if there is no evidence of impingement or there continues to be a question of viability with these maneuvers, the standard course of action is to perform bipolar exclusion.[4] One could consider proceeding with the operation using alternative conduit such as colon or jejunum, taking into account the total operative time that has passed and any bowel edema from intraoperative fluid administration, as well as the hemodynamic stability of the patient. Unstable patients should always be managed with resection of the ischemic tissue and exclusion, and in cases of severe instability, may be left in discontinuity with formalization of the esophagostomy and gastrostomy and jejunostomy 24 to 48 hours later once adequately resuscitated. An alternative to classic bipolar exclusion in patients with questionable conduit viability but without frank necrosis was described by Oezcelik and colleagues in 2009, in which the conduit is brought into the neck either substernally or in the typical posterior mediastinal position, but no anastomosis is made, instead creating a cervical esophagostomy and allowing a 90-day period for the conduit to declare itself—if it remains viable after this period, the anastomosis can be created via a neck incision.[6,35] This technique was performed in 37 patients, with 35/37 undergoing formalized reconstruction, and all of those 35 healing without any leak or necrosis, demonstrating the feasibility of this method.[35]

Patient Outcomes

As previously mentioned, at the extreme end of the spectrum of ischemic complications, frank gastric conduit necrosis carries a mortality rate of up to 90%. However, for those who do survive this complication or for those who have less severe manifestations of ischemia, the risk of additional complications, as well as the effect on mortality remains. For patients managed with exclusion, there is a subset that never achieves gastrointestinal continuity, often due to poor nutrition status or other comorbidities rendering the risk of an even more extensive, complex operation too great. For those that do undergo reconnection, the same operative risks of the initial procedure remain, often cited at higher frequencies due to increased complexity of the operation, and in cases of colonic or jejunal interposition in particular, rates of leak and ischemic complications are inherently higher. For those that survive ischemic complications without the takedown of their conduit, there remain increased rates of anastomotic stricture formation, postop atrial fibrillation, ventricular arrhythmias, deep vein thrombosis, pneumonia, empyema, acute respiratory distress syndrome, reintubation and prolonged respiratory failure, sepsis, and renal failure.[6,11] Formation of conduit-airway fistula has also been described, particularly in relation to endoscopic stent placement. The effect on short- and long-term mortality must also be considered. Specifically for those with anastomotic leak, which is perhaps the most common of these ischemic complications, there has been observed an increased 30-day mortality (7.2% vs 3.1% for patients with vs without), exacerbated in those requiring invasive surgical treatment for the leak (ie, uncontained), then cited at 11.6%.[11] This risk may extend beyond the perioperative period as well. In a study looking at mortality in post-esophagectomy patients at 60 months, there was a mean survival reduction of 4.2 months in those whose course had been complicated by leak. This long-term effect, particularly for cancer patients, is posited to be some combination of increased levels of inflammatory cytokines—some of which correlate with tumor growth—and delays in adjuvant treatment while the leak heals and due to malnutrition or deconditioning as a result of the leak and its associated complications. Finally, such complications have an impact on the patient's length of stay, overall costs, and quality of life.[36–40]

SUMMARY

Ischemic complications of the conduit following esophagectomy exist on a spectrum, from submucosal ischemia without disruption of gastrointestinal continuity to frank necrosis and mediastinal contamination with sepsis. These complications affect patients in terms of hospital costs, survival, and quality of life. Understanding the physiologic and anatomic basis for these complications and the mechanisms by which to prevent, diagnose, and treat them is vital for thoracic and foregut surgeons to minimize morbidity and mortality following esophagectomy.

CLINICS CARE POINTS

- Esophagectomy carries a morbidity of 66% at 30 days, with ramifications of conduit ischemia often being the most significant. Anastomotic leak is estimated at 11.4%, with frank conduit necrosis cited at 1% to 3%.
- In addition to meticulous operative technique, avoidance of hypotension, and

appropriate conduit decompression in the perioperative period, preoperative ischemic conditioning of the gastric conduit may benefit high-risk individuals.

- Diagnosis of ischemic complications rely on thr compiled clinical and laboratory data, with imaging or endoscopy used to confirm. CRP, trends, in particular, has shown some promise. While some advocate for screening for leaks at variable times within the first postoperative week with imaging, others argue this can be falsely reassuring as leaks may manifest up to 2 weeks postoperatively. Recent data suggest that CT chest may be more sensitive than traditional esophagram in detecting leaks and give additional information (drainable collections, etc.).

- Management of ischemic complications varies depending on the manifestations, with submucosal ischemia or pinhole leaks often controlled with conservative measures (limited PO intake, antibiotics), with more severe leaks requiring exclusion with a stent or EndoVac therapy with possible additional procedures to facilitate drainage. On the extreme end, complete conduit necrosis with sepsis requires prompt source control with takedown and resection of the conduit and bipolar exclusion.

- Patients with gastric conduit ischemia have increased mortality. Patients with anastomotic leaks have an estimated 30-day mortality of 7.2%, compared to those without leaks of 3.1%, while at 60-month follow-up, those with leaks had a mean reduction in survival of 4.2 months. For those with gastric conduit necrosis, mortality reaches up to 90%.

DISCLOSURE

The authors have nothing to disclose.

REFERENCES

1. Barbaro A, Eldredge TA, Shenfine J. Diagnosing anastomotic leak post-esophagectomy: a systematic review. Dis Esophagus 2021;34:1–15.
2. Yeung JC. Management of Complications After Esophagectomy. Thorac Surg Clin 2020;30:359–66.
3. Low DE, Alderson D, Cecconello I, et al. International Consensus on Standardization of Data Collection for Complications Associated With Esophagectomy: Esophagectomy Complications Consensus Group (ECCG). Ann Surg 2015;262(2):286–94.
4. Athanasiou A, Hennessy M, Spartalis E, et al. Conduit necrosis following esophagectomy: An

up-to-date literature review. World J Gastrointest Surg 2019;11(3):155–68.

5. Cassivi SD. Leaks, Strictures, and Necrosis: A Review of Anastomotic Complications Following Esophagectomy. Semin Thorac Cardiovasc Surg 2004;16(2):124–32.

6. Dickinson KJ, Blackmon SH. Management of Conduit Necrosis Following Esophagectomy. Thorac Surg Clin 2015;25:461–70.

7. Fabbi M, Hagens ERC, van Berge Henegouwen MI, et al. Anastomotic leakage after esophagectomy for esophageal cancer: definitions, diagnostics, and treatment. Dis Esophagus 2021;34:1–14.

8. Lainas P, Fuks D, Gaujoux S, et al. Preoperative imaging and prediction of oesophageal conduit necrosis after oesophagectomy for cancer. BJS 2017;104: 1346–54.

9. Ozawa S, Koyanagi K, Ninomiya Y, et al. Postoperative complications of minimally invasive esophagectomy for esophageal cancer. Ann Gastroenterol Surg 2020;4:126–34.

10. Junemann-Ramirez M, Awan MY, Khan ZM, et al. Anastomotic leakage post-esophagogastrectomy for esophageal carcinoma: retrospective analysis of predictive factors, management and influence on longterm survival in a high volume centre. Eur J Cardio Thorac Surg 2005;27:3–7.

11. Kassis ES, Kosinski AS, Ross Jr P, et al. Predictors of anastomotic leak after esophagectomy: an analysis of the society of thoracic surgeons general thoracic database. Ann Thorac Surg 2013;96(6): 1919–26.

12. van Kooten RT, Voeten DM, Steyerberg EW, et al. Patient-Related Prognostic Factors for Anastomotic Leakage, Major Complications, and Short-Term Mortality Following Esophagectomy for Cancer: A Systematic Review and Meta-Analyses. Ann Surg Oncol 2022;29:1358–73.

13. Nederlof N, Slaman AE, van Hagen P, et al. Using the Comprehensive Complication Index to Assess the Impact of Neoadjuvant Chemoradiotherapy on Complication Severity After Esophagectomy for Cancer. Ann Surg Oncol 2016;23:3964–71.

14. Levy RM, Trivedi D, Luketich JD. Minimally Invasive Esophagectomy. Surg Clin N Am 2012;92:1265–85.

15. Groth SS, Burt BM. Minimally invasive esophagectomy: Direction of the art. J Thorac Cardiovasc Surg 2021;162:701–4.

16. Markar SR, Arya S, Karthikesalingam A, et al. Technical Factors that Affect Anastomotic Integrity Following Esophagectomy: Systematic Review and Meta-analysis. Ann Surg Oncol 2013;20:4274–81.

17. Till BM, Grenda TR, Olugbenga OT, et al. Robotic Minimally Invasive Esophagectomy. Thorac Surg Clin 2023;33:81–8.

18. Nederlof N, Tilanus HW, Khe Tran TC, et al. End-to-End Versus End-to-Side Esophagogastrostomy After Esophageal Cancer Resection: A Prospective Randomized Study. Ann Surg 2011;254(2): 226–33.

19. Lu M, Luketich JD, Levy RM, et al. Anastomotic complications after esophagectomy: Influence of omentoplasty in propensity-weighted cohorts. J Thorac Cardiovasc Surg 2020;159:2096–105.

20. Chen L, Liu F, Wang K, et al. Omentoplasty in the prevention of anastomotic leakage after oesophagectomy: a meta-analysis. Eur J Surg Oncol 2014; 40(12):1635–40.

21. Yuan Y, Zeng X, Hu Y, et al. Omentoplasty for oesophagogastrostomy after oesophagectomy. Cochrane Database Syst Rev 2014;10:CD008446.

22. van der Sluis PC, van der Horst S, May AM, et al. Robot-assisted Minimally Invasive Thoracolaparoscopic Esophagectomy Versus Open Transthoracic Esophagectomy for Resectable Esophageal Cancer: A Randomized Control Trial. Ann Surg 2019; 269(4):621–30.

23. Walsh KJ, Zhang H, Tan KS, et al. Use of vasopressors during esophagectomy is not associated with increased risk of anastomotic leak. Dis Esophagus 2021;34(4):doaa090.

24. Aiolfi A, Bona D, Bonitta G, et al. Effect of gastric ischemic conditioning prior to esophagectomy: systematic review and meta-analysis. Updates Surg 2023;75:1633–43.

25. de Groot E, Schiffmann LM, van der Veen A, et al. Laparoscopic ischemic conditioning prior esophagectomy in selected patients: the ISCON trial. Dis Esophagus 2023;36(11):1–7.

26. Hölscher AH, Schneider PM, Gutschow C, et al. Laparoscopic ischemic conditioning of the stomach for esophageal replacement. Ann Surg 2007;245(2): 241–6.

27. Mils K, Miró M, Farran L, et al. A pilot randomized controlled trial on the utility of gastric conditioning in the prevention of esophagogastric anastomotic leak after Ivor Lewis esophagectomy. The APIL_ 2013 Trial. Int Surg J 2022;106:106921.

28. Schröder W, Hölscher AH, Bludau M, et al. Ivor-Lewis Esophagectomy With and Without Laparoscopic Conditioning of the Gastric Conduit. World J Surg 2010;34(4):738–43.

29. Dalton BGA, Ali AA, Crandall M, et al. Near infrared perfusion assessment of gastric conduit during minimally invasive Ivor Lewis esophagectomy. Am J Surg 2018;216:524–7.

30. Veeramootoo D, Parameswaran R, Krishnadas R, et al. Classification and early recognition of gastric conduit failure after minimally invasive esophagectomy. Surg Endosc 2009;23:2110–6.

31. Shoji Y, Takeuchi H, Fukuda K, et al. Air Bubble Sign: A New Screening Method for Anastomotic Leakage After Esophagectomy for Esophageal Cancer. Ann Surg Oncol 2018;25:1061–8.

32. Freeman RK, Vyverberg A, Ascioti AJ. Esophageal Stent Placement for the Treatment of Acute Intrathoracic Anastomotic Leak After Esophagectomy. Ann Thorac Surg 2011;92:204–8.

33. Hallit R, Calmels M, Chaput U, et al. Endoscopic management of anastomotic leak after esophageal or gastric resection for malignancy: a multicenter experience. Therap Adv Gastroenterol 2021;14. 17562848211932823.

34. Blackmon SH, Correa AM, Skoracki R, et al. Ann Thorac Surg 2012;94:1104–13.

35. Oezcelik A, Banki F, DeMeester SR, et al. Delayed esophagogastrostomy: a safe strategy for management of patients with ischemic gastric conduit at the time of esophagectomy. J Am Coll Surg 2009; 208:1030–4.

36. Aiolfi A, Griffiths EA, Sozzi A, et al. Effect of Anastomotic Leak on Long-Term Survival After Esophagectomy: Multivariate Meta-analysis and Restricted Mean Survival Times Examination. Ann Surg Oncol 2023;30: 5564–72.

37. Crestanello JA, Deschamps C, Cassivi SD, et al. Selective management of intrathoracic anastomotic leak after esophagectomy. J Thorac Cardiovasc Surg 2005;129:254–60.

38. Linder G, Hedberg J, Björck M, et al. Dis Esophagus 2017;30:143–9.

39. Ubels S, Verstegen M, Klarenbeek B, et al. Severity of oEsophageal Anastomotic Leak in patients after oesophagectomy: the SEAL score. BJS 2022;109:864–71.

40. van der Veen A, Schiffmann LM, de Groot EM, et al. The ISCON-trial protocol: laparoscopic ischemic conditioning prior to esophagectomy in patients with esophageal cancer and arterial calcifications. BMC Cancer 2022;22(1):144.

UNITED STATES POSTAL SERVICE ® Statement of Ownership, Management, and Circulation
(All Periodicals Publications Except Requester Publications)

1. Publication Title	2. Publication Number	3. Filing Date
THORACIC SURGERY CLINICS	013 – 26	9/18/2024

4. Issue Frequency	5. Number of Issues Published Annually	6. Annual Subscription Price
FEB, MAY, AUG, NOV	4	$434.00

7. Complete Mailing Address of Known Office of Publication (Not printer) (Street, city, county, state, and ZIP+4®)

ELSEVIER INC.
230 Park Avenue, Suite 800
New York, NY 10169

Contact Person
Malathi Samayan

Telephone (Include area code)
91-44-4299-4507

8. Complete Mailing Address of Headquarters or General Business Office of Publisher (Not printer)

ELSEVIER INC.
230 Park Avenue, Suite 800
New York, NY 10169

9. Full Names and Complete Mailing Addresses of Publisher, Editor, and Managing Editor (Do not leave blank)

Publisher (Name and complete mailing address)

Dolores Meloni, ELSEVIER INC.
1600 JOHN F KENNEDY BLVD. SUITE 1600
PHILADELPHIA, PA 19103-2899

Editor (Name and complete mailing address)

JOHN VASSALLO, ELSEVIER INC.
1600 JOHN F KENNEDY BLVD. SUITE 1600
PHILADELPHIA, PA 19103-2899

Managing Editor (Name and complete mailing address)

PATRICK MANLEY, ELSEVIER INC.
1600 JOHN F KENNEDY BLVD. SUITE 1600
PHILADELPHIA, PA 19103-2899

10. Owner (Do not leave blank. If the publication is owned by a corporation, give the name and address of the corporation immediately followed by the names and addresses of all stockholders owning or holding 1 percent or more of the total amount of stock. If not owned by a corporation, give the names and addresses of the individual owners. If owned by a partnership or other unincorporated firm, give its name and address as well as those of each individual owner. If the publication is published by a nonprofit organization, give its name and address.)

Full Name	Complete Mailing Address
WHOLLY OWNED SUBSIDIARY OF REED/ELSEVIER, US HOLDINGS	1600 JOHN F KENNEDY BLVD. SUITE 1600 PHILADELPHIA, PA 19103-2899

11. Known Bondholders, Mortgagees, and Other Security Holders Owning or Holding 1 Percent or More of Total Amount of Bonds, Mortgages, or Other Securities. If none, check box ▶ ☐ None

Full Name	Complete Mailing Address
N/A	

12. Tax Status (For completion by nonprofit organizations authorized to mail at nonprofit rates) (Check one)
The purpose, function, and nonprofit status of this organization and the exempt status for federal income tax purposes:
☒ Has Not Changed During Preceding 12 Months
☐ Has Changed During Preceding 12 Months (Publisher must submit explanation of change with this statement)

PS Form **3526**, July 2014 [Page 1 of 4 (see instructions page 4)] PSN: 7530-01-000-9931 PRIVACY NOTICE: See our privacy policy on www.usps.com.

---

13. Publication Title	14. Issue Date for Circulation Data Below
THORACIC SURGERY CLINICS	AUGUST 2024

15. Extent and Nature of Circulation			Average No. Copies Each Issue During Preceding 12 Months	No. Copies of Single Issue Published Nearest to Filing Date
a. Total Number of Copies (Net press run)			144	139
b. Paid Circulation (By Mail and Outside the Mail)	(1)	Mailed Outside-County Paid Subscriptions Stated on PS Form 3541 (Include paid distribution above nominal rate, advertiser's proof copies, and exchange copies)	87	89
	(2)	Mailed In-County Paid Subscriptions Stated on PS Form 3541 (Include paid distribution above nominal rate, advertiser's proof copies, and exchange copies)	0	0
	(3)	Paid Distribution Outside the Mails Including Sales Through Dealers and Carriers, Street Vendors, Counter Sales, and Other Paid Distribution Outside USPS®	42	38
	(4)	Paid Distribution by Other Classes of Mail Through the USPS (e.g., First-Class Mail®)	12	9
c. Total Paid Distribution (Sum of 15b (1), (2), (3), and (4))		▶	141	136
d. Free or Nominal Rate Distribution (By Mail and Outside the Mail)	(1)	Free or Nominal Rate Outside-County Copies included on PS Form 3541	3	3
	(2)	Free or Nominal Rate In-County Copies Included on PS Form 3541	0	0
	(3)	Free or Nominal Rate Copies Mailed at Other Classes Through the USPS (e.g., First-Class Mail)	0	0
	(4)	Free or Nominal Rate Distribution Outside the Mail (Carriers or other means)	0	0
e. Total Free or Nominal Rate Distribution (Sum of 15d (1), (2), (3) and (4))		▶	3	3
f. Total Distribution (Sum of 15c and 15e)		▶	144	139
g. Copies not Distributed (See Instructions to Publishers #4 (page #3))		▶	0	0
h. Total (Sum of 15f and g)		▶	144	139
i. Percent Paid (15c divided by 15f times 100)		▶	98.09%	97.84%

* If you are claiming electronic copies, go to line 16 on page 3. If you are not claiming electronic copies, skip to line 17 on page 3.

16. Electronic Copy Circulation	Average No. Copies Each Issue During Preceding 12 Months	No. Copies of Single Issue Published Nearest to Filing Date
a. Paid Electronic Copies ▶		
b. Total Paid Print Copies (Line 15c) + Paid Electronic Copies (Line 16a) ▶		
c. Total Print Distribution (Line 15f) + Paid Electronic Copies (Line 16a) ▶		
d. Percent Paid (Both Print & Electronic Copies) (16b divided by 16c × 100) ▶		

☒ I certify that 50% of all my distributed copies (electronic and print) are paid above a nominal price.

17. Publication of Statement of Ownership

☒ If the publication is a general publication, publication of this statement is required. Will be printed in the _NOVEMBER 2024_ issue of this publication.   ☐ Publication not required.

18. Signature and Title of Editor, Publisher, Business Manager, or Owner

Malathi Samayan

Malathi Samayan - Distribution Controller

Date 9/18/2024

I certify that all information furnished on this form is true and complete. I understand that anyone who furnishes false or misleading information on this form or who omits material or information requested on the form may be subject to criminal sanctions (including fines and imprisonment) and/or civil sanctions (including civil penalties).

PS Form **3526**, July 2014 (Page 2 of 4)   PRIVACY NOTICE: See our privacy policy on www.usps.com

Moving?

Make sure your subscription moves with you!

To notify us of your new address, find your **Clinics Account Number** (located on your mailing label above your name), and contact customer service at:

Email: journalscustomerservice-usa@elsevier.com

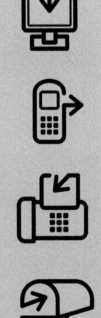

800-654-2452 (subscribers in the U.S. & Canada)
314-447-8871 (subscribers outside of the U.S. & Canada)

Fax number: 314-447-8029

Elsevier Health Sciences Division
Subscription Customer Service
3251 Riverport Lane
Maryland Heights, MO 63043

*To ensure uninterrupted delivery of your subscription, please notify us at least 4 weeks in advance of move.